Child Taming
How to Manage Children in Dental Practice

Quintessentials of Dental Practice – 9
Paediatric Dentistry/Orthodontics - 1

Child Taming

How to Manage Children in Dental Practice

By
Barbara L Chadwick
Marie Thérèse Hosey

Editor-in-Chief: Nairn H F Wilson
Editor Paediatric Dentistry/Orthodontics: Marie Thérèse Hosey

Quintessence Publishing Co. Ltd.

London, Berlin, Chicago, Copenhagen, Paris, Milan, Barcelona, Istanbul, São Paulo, Tokyo, New Dehli, Moscow, Prague, Warsaw

British Library Cataloguing in Publication Data

Chadwick, Barbara L.
   Child taming : how to manage children in dental practice. – (Quintessentials of dental
   practice ; 9. Paediatric dentistry/orthodontics ; 1)
   1. Pedodontics 2. Children – Dental care
   I. Title II. Hosey, Marie Thérèse
   617.6'45

ISBN 1850970629

ISBN 1-85097-062-9

Acknowledgements

Dr Andrew Makin, Consultant Anaesthetist, for the paediatric anatomy and physiology; Caroline Campbell and Alison Cairns for their wonderful contribution to both the clinical photographs and commentary on the developing text; and finally, Jason Leitch, Graeme Wright and Ed Hosey for their help with the proof-reading.

A special thanks to Gail Drake in the Photography Department, Glasgow Dental Hospital and School and Jo Griffiths, Dental Illustration Unit, Dental School, Cardiff and finally and especially to all the children who agreed to model for us.

Foreword

The frightened, fractious, four-year-old, first-attendance child; the fussing, fraught, dentally frightened mother:

"Sweetheart, it's OK! The dentist - the one in the white coat - won't really hurt you. The injection will be worth it to get rid of that nasty toothache. Just hold tight on to the chair."

How well do you manage this sort of situation? Can you confidently sense what the child is thinking? How will she react to your approach? Is your practice child friendly? And are you up to date on consent, conscious sedation, and when and how to refer for treatment under general anaesthesia?

Child Taming: How to Manage Children in Dental Practice - the ninth volume in the Quintessentials of Dental Practice series has been written to help the busy practitioner address these questions, and many more, for the best management of child patients. Possibly the nearest thing you will get to a ready reckoner to assess the level of anxiety of a child patient and provide advice for effective care. Well-presented (as you expect of Quintessence Publishing) and neatly packaged, in an easy-to-read style (as you would expect of the Quintessentials of Dental Practice series): an attractive package.

Have you met the kids in the cartoons? If you haven't, they are bound to turn up in your practice sooner or later. Will you be prepared for them? If in doubt, this book is for you.

Nairn Wilson
Editor-in-Chief

Preface

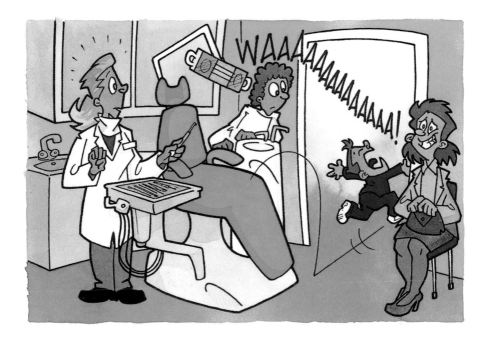

The dental surgery is an alien place to a child. Strangers in crisp uniforms inhabit the inner sanctum, whilst other grown-ups sit or pace around waiting, looking weary or worried or frightened. There are strange smells, clinical colours and posters on the walls reminiscent of visiting the school sick bay, and shining, sharp-looking instruments lying out ready for use. Within the many drawers and cupboards other things are hidden ... It is rumoured at school that dentists hurt. Grandparents have been telling some scary stories recently and parents had warned that you end up at the dentist when too much sugar is eaten. There are rules here that only the dentist and perhaps a few parents understand, but the child has still to learn them.

It is hardly surprising that dentistry provokes apprehension in children but there is no doubt that successfully managing children presents both the greatest challenge and the greatest reward for a dentist. This book is less about child taming and more about training the dental team and parents how to work together to ensure that a child's visit to the dentist is a pleasurable experience.

Childhood apprehension about dentistry is not limited to children in the United Kingdom. A study of 3,200 children in eight European countries (including the United Kingdom) found 35% of five-year-olds and 21% of 12-year-olds were fearful before visiting the dentist. Interestingly, the parents of 32% of five-year-olds and 30% of 12-year-olds across Europe reported that they too were fearful before a dental visit. This data suggests that anxiety is so prevalent that it should be considered normal. Indeed, making the assumption that the majority of patients may be suffering from some degree of anxiety might remind the dentist and their team to approach children, especially, in a sympathetic manner -- thereby enhancing the likelihood of a successful introduction to life-long dental care.

In this book we hope to give family dentists the keys to successful child management by showing how to:
- create a child-friendly atmosphere
- co-ordinate the whole dental team
- communicate with children and their families
- create a treatment plan conducive to child care
- utilise behavioural management techniques
- decide when and how to use conscious sedation and general anaesthesia
- link with wider specialist and community services.

Contents

Chapter 1
Introducing the Children

Aim

In this chapter the stages of child development and individual personality will be reviewed, and the potential impact of these upon providing dental care explored.

Outcome

Reading this chapter should enable the whole dental team to take a child-centred approach towards the delivery of paediatric dental care (Fig 1-1).

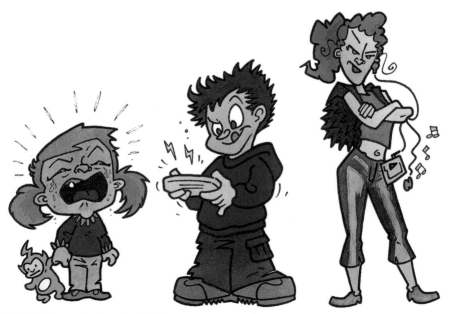

Fig 1-1 Introducing the children.

Introduction

Although each child is an individual, there are well-recognised stages of child development that may give an appropriate framework to approach child management. These are outlined in Table 1-1. Indeed, an understanding of normal child development is essential for anyone who wants to work success-

Table 1-1 **Stages of child development**

2-year-old	GDP
Self-centred, solitary, easily frustrated, easily distracted and completely dependent on adults. Attention span of 1–5 minutes. Concentrates on one thing at a time. Lives in the present. *Favourite word: No!*	Avoid asking questions which can have a "no" answer such as "Would you like me to ... ?" Keep appointment times short. Invite a parent but not other siblings into the surgery. Concentrate only on the child and avoid interruptions from parents or other staff. Avoid sudden movements.
3-year-old	
Exuberant, independent, imitative of adult behaviour, curious, imaginative. Attention span of 4–8 minutes. Eager to please. *Favourite word: Why?*	Gain attention by arousing curiosity, describe procedures to the child and ask them to add their own description. Let them "help". Be positive (e.g. "It's better if you ... " rather than "don't do that").
4-year-old	
Dominant, bossy, impatient, insistent. Grasps simple reasoning, is willing to accept change. Enjoys variety.	Engage the child's "help". Explain simple procedures (e.g. "The filling doesn't stick if the tooth gets wet"). Keep working steadily, avoid pauses, don't loose control.
5-year-old	
Poised, self-confident, aware of rules, likes to act grown-up, less combative, accepts authority. Proud of their possessions. Has feelings that are easily hurt.	Show interest in possessions /clothes. Appeal to their vanity (e.g. "A dirty tooth ... I'll clean it and put a pretty silver filling in it"; "I need you to help me fix it". Give praise. Should be able to use a hand signal properly

Based on Lowrey, Growth and Development of Children, 6th edn. (1974).

fully with children. Once you understand the child's level of emotional development and maturity you can more easily predict, and correctly interpret, some of their behaviour as it manifests in the surgery. Similarly, it becomes easier to set reasonable, achievable goals for each child. Understanding what to expect of a child in relation to what that child is able to do in life will make the dental team feel less stressed the next time they encounter a "pre-cooperative" two-year-old, belligerent adolescent or precocious primary school child (Fig 1-2).

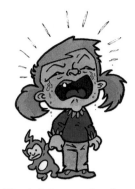

Fig 1-2 A pre-schooler.

Milestones in Child Development

Pre-school children (two to four years)

The term "the terrible twos" exists because this age group can be awkward to deal with (ask the parent of any two-year-old). The term "pre-cooperative" describes them perfectly. They have limited communication skills, are very dependent on their parents and do not play or share with others well. When they do speak it is usually to say "No!" as this is their favourite word. Because they cannot express themselves verbally their common response to any upset is to cry. Their parents know that they cry when interrupted while playing, tired or hungry. However, the parents may themselves be stressed during a dental visit and it is important that they are helped to realise that tears for this group are often a normal part of the circumstances, not a sign that something is going wrong. To be successful with this group, the dentist must be quick (an attention span of less than five minutes is normal) and make use of the parents on whom the child remains dependent (see further, Chapter 2).

Three-year-olds

The three-year-old likes to please you but is still very attached to his or her parents. Although they are beginning to be able to communicate, tears are not too far below the surface, so, again, you need to use the parents to help you. This fear of strangers (separation anxiety) is strongest in the under-twos, but remains common until about the age of five. Children are beginning to explore the world, so expect them to ask "Why?" in response to almost any request. Three-year-olds respond well to colourful descriptions and stories that capture their imagination. They also like to copy adult behaviour, which can be to your advantage. By the age of three, they can concentrate for up to eight minutes, so you still need to be slick (Fig 1-3).

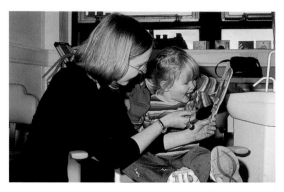

Fig 1-3 Capture the pre-school child's imagination.

Four-year-olds
By the age of four, children are becoming more self-determining and begin to try to impose their will. They are able to interact in small groups and start to develop independent skills. It may be possible for the dental nurse to engage the child while you speak to the parent. Four-year-old children understand how to use "Thank you" and "Please". They often express their independence by rejecting previously established patterns of behaviour. For example, they no longer want to have their teeth brushed, they want to do it themselves. But they lack the ability to do it well. Parents and carers may sometimes allow this rather than have a battle every night with the toothbrush. Let parents know that this is normal and not just happening to their child.

In other words, by the age of four, children are "potentially cooperative". In fact, most children who find dentistry difficult fall into this group. For each developmental stage you need to find the best approach.

The school child

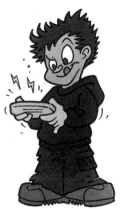

Once children start school they require less parental support. By the age of five they respond well to flattery and like to know that they are performing well. They take pride in their possessions and like to show them to you. They also begin to relinquish comfort objects. Constant positive feedback works well, but they still find it hard to concentrate for long periods. They can recognize simple concepts, but you must use language

Fig 1-4 Schoolboy.

they will understand (Fig 1-4). They are still egocentric and inflexible, finding it difficult to identify with a point of view other than their own. This single-mindedness remains until around the age of seven (Fig 1-5).

By the age of seven, children can determine which messages deserve their attention and which they can ignore. They usually have sufficient co-ordination to brush their own teeth, but may lack the motivation to carry it out. From seven to eleven years of age, children begin to apply logical reasoning – they are able to understand an alternative view and to consider different aspects of a situation.

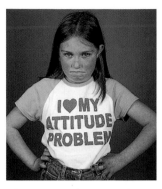

Fig 1-5 An alternate view?

Adolescents

Adolescents become increasingly independent of their parents. There are major emotional, physical and hormonal changes during the teenage years and for many young people these changes can be perplexing. Adolescents may be moody and can be very sensitive to criticism, so comments about their oral health need to be delivered with care. They require support and reassurance, but may be difficult to motivate unless there are acute problems, as they are usually firmly fixed in the present. They are, however, able to consider difficult abstract problems and to determine the effects of different actions (Fig 1-6).

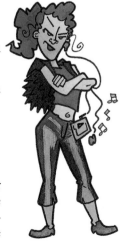

The Relationship between Age and Behaviour in the Dental Surgery

Children's clinical behaviour may be characterised in three ways (Fig 1-7):
- cooperative
- potentially cooperative
- lacking cooperative ability ("pre-cooperative").

Behaviour-management techniques are appropriate for cooperative and potentially cooperative children. The term "cooperative" is self-explanatory, while "potentially cooperative" is preferred to "uncooperative". The "uncooperative" label is frequently applied to children

Fig 1-6 Teenager.

5

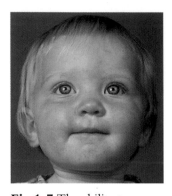 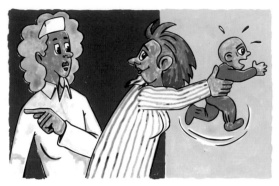

Fig 1-7 The ability to cooperate is dependent on age.

Fig 1-8 Dental treatment for the pre-cooperative
child.

who have experienced difficulty in the dental surgery, sometimes on only
one occasion. The term implies that a child is deliberately difficult or obstruc-
tive, which is rarely the case (Fig 1-8).

"Pre-cooperative"

The "pre-cooperative" child is a child who lacks cooperative ability. This
includes the very young child with whom communication cannot yet be
established (even though they may be "potentially cooperative" when they
mature). Children with specific disabilities (with whom cooperation in the
usual manner may never be achieved) also fall into this category. Both groups
need different approaches, which may include general anaesthesia.

The Effect of Personality on Behaviour

Introvert versus extrovert

While developmental stages are useful in identifying how children change
as they grow, they are still individuals, and not every child of the same age
reacts in the same way. These differences can be attributed to personality
variables. Personality is hard to define but it has been suggested that it is made
up of stable internal factors that are relatively constant over time. Some char-
acteristics, like shyness, may be more obvious at certain stages, such as adolescents dealing with their developing bodies. But it is also possible to identify individuals who are shy or outgoing. These are sometimes referred to as
"introverts" or "extroverts". While these "internal" factors influence our
behaviours, external circumstances may exert a powerful effect also. It is
common to be told that a quiet, shy child in our surgery is completely dif-

ferent at home. The out-of-character behaviour may be symptomatic of anxiety (Fig 1-9).

One's character determines how a child will respond to a new situation. Some respond positively (by smiling and getting on with the challenge), others are more negative (fussing and pulling away). Indeed, studies have shown that the latter group is more often referred to specialists in dental centres for treatment, perhaps because the children require more time to adapt. Where the pulling away is accompanied by clinging to a parent, we sometimes suggest that they are "young for their age" – that is, they require more parental support than we deem necessary. Such children are challenged by new situations, both dental and non-dental. They benefit from

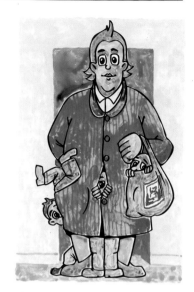

Fig 1-9 Some children are challenged by new situations.

a gradual introduction to dental care and continue to require this gradual approach when a new procedure is introduced.

Locus of control

Individuals have different beliefs about how they can influence events. This is termed their "locus of control". Those who believe they can control what happens to them are termed "internals". Those who believe that what happens is down to chance are termed "externals". This belief system is significant in determining preventive health care as the "internal" is far more likely to take preventive actions and to take responsibility for their own care. In contrast, the "external" believes that good oral health is a matter of luck or can be influenced by someone else (a dentist, for example), but is something they cannot control themselves. This group needs much more motivation and reinforcement.

Interestingly, a patient's locus of control is important when giving information. Children with an internal locus of control need a lot of specific information about the treatment that they are to undergo, as it helps them to feel in control. If they are given general information without detail, they are more likely to feel anxious. For the child with an external locus of control the opposite is true: he or she responds best to an outline of what is required. Long, detailed information is more likely to increase their anxiety levels.

Trait anxiety

Some individuals are inherently more anxious than others – this is termed "trait anxiety". For some very anxious patients their dental difficulties are mirrored by similar fears in many settings and they may be prone to excessive worry about many aspects of their lives, especially if an element of failure is possible. The thing to remember with trait anxiety is that it is stable over time. Such patients are likely to be just as anxious at the review visit as they were to begin with. This can be frustrating for the clinician, but is also frustrating for your patient too. As they get older they can be embarrassed by their anxiety and need continuing support to help them control it.

Practical Tips

- Remember that the ability of a child to cooperate for dental treatment is dependent upon their stage of development.
- Toddlers <u>will</u> cry – so expect it!
- Pre-cooperative children simply lack the ability to cooperate, but they may improve as they mature.
- Personality and trait anxiety influence behaviour anxiety.

Further Reading

Freeman R. Psychodynamic theory of dental phobia. Brit Dent J 184;1988:170-172.

Lowrey GH, Growth and Development of Children. 6th edn. Chicago: Year Book Medical Publishers, Inc., 1974: 138-139.

Moore R, Brodsgard I, Birn H. Manifestations, acquisitions and diagnostic categories of dental fear in a self reported population. Behav Res Ther 29; 1991:51-60.

Wright G, Starkey PE, Gardener DE, Curzon MEJ. Child Management in Dentistry. Bristol: Wright, 1987.

Chapter 2
Child Taming I:
This Is What I See, Hear and Feel

Aim

This chapter will review how anxiety presents in the dental surgery, how to communicate with children and how to create a child-friendly environment.

Outcome

The dental team should be able to anticipate a child's reaction to the dental environment and procedures and, by so doing, be able to take simple, practical steps to avoid undesirable consequences (Fig 2-1).

Introduction

Once the level of emotional development and maturity is understood we can begin to predict how a child of any given age might behave. The next key to successful management is to correctly interpret anxiety-related behaviour when it becomes manifest in the surgery.

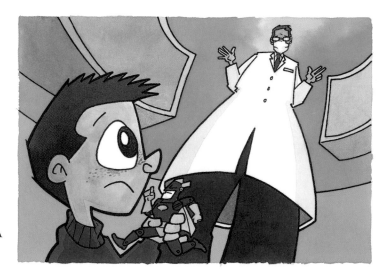

Fig 2-1 A child's-eye view.

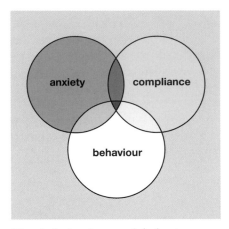

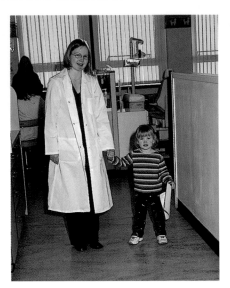

Fig 2-2 Anxiety and behaviour are interlinked in children.

Fig 2-3 Dentist and child.

Anxiety

We know that a toddler manifests only one reaction – crying – to deal with most "negative" situations. It should also be noted that fear of the unknown is widespread in young children. It is normal for younger children to report fear regardless of the anticipated treatment or even prior to their first dental visit (Fig 2-2).

For older children the situation is not so straightforward: they demonstrate anxiety in different ways, and while some signs are easy to spot, others are more subtle. Therefore, we will first explore the reasons for dental anxiety in children and then how anxiety manifests itself, before examining how to deal with it. Anxiety is common and the consequences of anxiety are dependent on the age of the child.

Common dental anxieties in children
The most common dental anxieties amongst children can be attributed to fear of the unknown and the lack of control that dental procedures can impose (Fig 2-3).

Fear of the unknown
For some patients, not knowing what is going to happen is a major component in their anxiety. This is demonstrated by the patient who is anxious

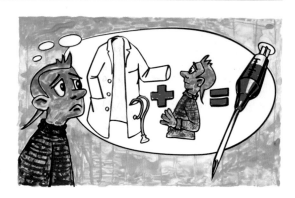

Fig 2-4 Fear of the unex-
pected.

when you first meet them but who overcomes their worries when they get
to know you. They appear happy and relaxed in the surgery until you suggest that they need some treatment. At this point they revert to their anxious state because they do not know what this entails.

One variation on this theme is knowing that something will happen but not
knowing when. The classic example is the patient who was once given a
local anaesthetic without warning and now expects one every time you move
a hand out of their line of sight. For many patients, the unknown is a major
source of concern and they require information and explanations in advance
to allow them to prepare (Fig 2-4).

Lack of control
Lying in a dental chair may produce a feeling of helplessness for many patients.
Coupled with an inability to talk to the dentist, because of a mouth full of instruments, this can translate to a feeling like a lack of control. The patient may
believe they have no way to interrupt proceedings if something goes wrong.

Factors that influence dental anxiety in children
Dental anxiety is common but clearly not experienced by all children. It is
often suggested that a negative dental experience will lead to dental anxiety,
but some patients are anxious without ever visiting the dentist while others
become happy and compliant patients despite unfortunate introductions to
dental care. Clearly, the aetiology of dental anxiety is not straightforward.

Factors associated with dental anxiety include:
- the attitude of parents towards dental treatment
- the child's medical and dental experience

- the dental experience of friends and siblings
- the type of preparation at home prior to the dental visit
- the child's own perception that something is wrong with his or her teeth.

Parental attitude
The importance of maternal anxiety has been recognised for over 100 years and the relationship between maternal anxiety and child behaviour is well documented. While a definite relationship between the child's behaviour and their anxiety as assessed by the mother has been shown at all ages, the effect is greatest on children under four years of age. In other words, parents who are anxious of dental treatment tend to have children who are anxious too.

Medical and dental experience
Children who are uncooperative or anxious during a dental visit are more likely to have experienced traumatic or painful dental procedures in the past than those who behave well. However, not all patients who have had pain during dental treatment become anxious. Bernstein and colleagues present data that suggest that the dentist is a key variable in the development of dental anxiety. They took groups of university students with either high fear or low fear towards dentistry and examined essays written on childhood experiences of dental procedures. In the high-fear group 42% had experienced pain during a visit but many of them also reported their dentists to be cold and uncaring, or used similar negative descriptions. Only 17% of the low-anxiety group had experienced pain but for this group the dentist was more likely to be described as careful, caring or friendly. This suggests that an empathic approach may overcome the long-term effects of pain.

Previous unpleasant medical experiences may also affect a child's subsequent ability to accept dentistry. However, it is the emotional quality of the episode not the number of visits that is significant. Children who have had positive medical experiences may be less apprehensive in the dental surgery. Pain experienced during medical appointments, or at least the parents' beliefs about the pain experienced, has been found to correlate well with their child's behaviour in a dental setting.

The dental experiences of others ("vicarious learning")
Many people who are anxious concerning dental treatment have never had a bad dental experience themselves; for example, many children and adults who have never received a local injection expect it to hurt. Children in particular may learn from exaggerated playground stories but may also reflect the dental anxiety of their parents.

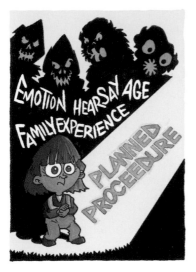

Fig 2-5 In the mind of the child.

Fig 2-6 Even happy toddlers will cry when separated from their mother.

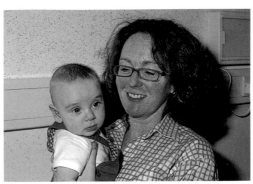

A child's awareness of dental problems

Children who attend a dentist for the first time and who know they have a dental problem (whatever it may be) tend to behave poorly. It has been suggested that transmission of maternal anxiety may be partially responsible. However, fear of pain is a common finding in children and may also be a significant factor (Fig 2-5).

A cursory look at these factors shows that children and their families may well be anxious before you ever meet them. Their introduction to your surgery can make it better or much worse. For example, the way the appointment is made will influence the parents, the parents anxieties will influence the child. The appearance of the staff and the reception area, the sounds, the smells that greet the patient all send messages, and the family are forming a view of your practice before they see you for the first time.

How children manifest anxiety

Toddlers

Toddlers are generally "pre-cooperative": they have very limited communication skills and few ways of expressing their anxiety and fears (Fig 2-6). When they feel unsure or threatened they try to escape and they usually do this by crying. Crying is an aversive stimulus that prompts the listener to act; that is, the parent intervenes to stop whatever is making the child cry.

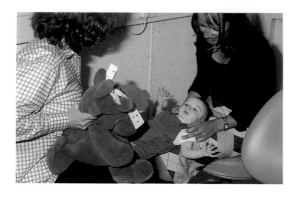

Fig 2-7 The baby or small child can still see her parent during the examination.

Toddlers cry for many reasons including:
- fear
- tiredness
- frustration
- pain
- when an activity is interrupted
- when separated from a parent
- when their nappy is damp.

So when you work with young children you should expect a few tears. The dental team needs to know how to deal with them and the family needs to be forewarned (Fig 2-7).
- Tell the parents that the child may cry when you examine them and that this is a normal reaction.
- Reassure the parents that the crying is a protest against being examined, not a sign of pain.
- Ask the parents to listen – most parents can detect the difference between their child's cry when frustrated and when in pain.
- Tell the parents that the crying will stop almost as soon as you finish.

Examining a young child is best undertaken when he or she is sitting on a parent's lap. This allows the dentist to examine the child easily while the parent can maintain eye contact with the child and hold his or her hands and feet. A parent's lap is far less threatening than a dental chair and a much easier position for an examination than trying to balance both parent and child on the dental chair.

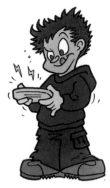

Fig 2-8 Is there such a thing as a "typical" schoolchild?.

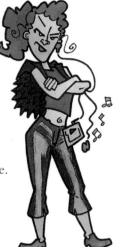

Fig 2-9 Adolescence.

School-age children

Children of around school age may show their anxiety by complaining of stomach pain or by frequently asking to go to the lavatory, whilst older children may complain of headache or dizziness and may fidget or stutter. However, not all children who are anxious will necessarily show their anxiety so do not be deceived by the child who appears to be compliant. Older children have more experience and have learned how to hide their fears and anxieties, as do adults. They have learned how they are supposed to behave in a dental surgery and this is what they manifest (Fig 2-8).

For example, a child who has learned what happens during an examination or restoration and who behaves well for these procedures may suddenly fail to cope when you do something new, like taking an impression. This is because they do not know what to expect or how to behave in a new situation. Their anxiety levels increase and they may even refuse to continue.

Adolescents

The adolescent years can be confusing: bodies begin to change; the young person will have near-adult intellectual abilities, but may lack adult knowledge and experience. During adolescence children start to distance themselves from their parents and may experiment with a variety of roles and behaviours before settling down. It is not unusual for many different hairstyles, colours, fashions and behaviours to manifest. The adolescent frequently complains that they are expected to behave as adults but not given adult freedoms. It is important that they be involved in decisions regarding their own care, unless they actively devolve the role to their parents (Fig 2-9).

Anxious adolescents may revert to younger behaviours by trying to escape. Alternatively they may show anxiety as rudeness or aggression. The parent who has been of assistance in the past may now be less helpful as the adolescent takes delight in disagreeing with them. Other adolescents may have become adept at hiding their anxiety. Some studies have shown that observing adults and adolescents in the waiting room before treatment may give a better indication of their anxiety than their behaviour in the surgery.

Communicating with Children

"I know you believe you understand what you think I said, but I am not sure you realise that what you heard is not what I meant". (MJ Geboy, Poem Attributed to the Religious Public Relations Council, 1985).

Communication is a balancing act and when and how you impart information is significant. This balancing act is at its most difficult when children are involved, as any information needs to be delivered to the child and to the parent as well. It is very easy to get sidetracked by a parent and to forget the child as a result. Ensure that the child is the centre of attention, while remembering to keep the parents appropriately involved (see also Chapter 4). Communication is a two-way process made up of three parts: words, tone, non-verbal. Surprisingly, the actual words are the smallest components (see Fig 2-10).

The message you think you are sending may not be the one the family is receiving. For young children, the words you use will have less impact than your tone of voice and the effect your words have on their parents. For older children, long explanations to the parents may use up their attention span or make them more anxious if they do not understand what you are saying.

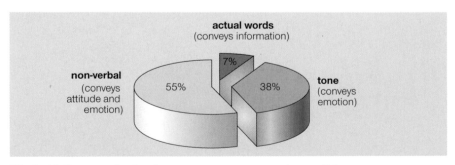

Fig 2-10 Communication is a two-way process made up of three parts.

Communication Pitfalls – The words we use
Verbal communication
Jargon

Dentistry has a language all of its own. It becomes second nature when talking with fellow professionals. When we are flustered or anxious it is very easy to lapse into jargon that has no meaning for the patient. As a result, the child misunderstands or becomes anxious because the treatment proposition sounds frightening.

Level

The words used need to be appropriate for the person you are talking to. Explanations given at the wrong level may be insulting, frightening or completely incomprehensible. This may seem hard if you need the child and the adult to understand. But remember, most parents will understand that you are trying to make things easier for their child and will appreciate your effort.

Listening

It is estimated that we listen at 25% of our potential, and our ability to listen decreases if we are anxious or awaiting treatment. This means that you may need to give some information in advance of the appointment to allow the family to prepare.

Retention

Fifty percent of information is forgotten within five minutes of leaving the surgery. It may be helpful to write down the critical messages or pieces of information for future reference.

Distortion

"Sugar-free" is recalled as "reduced-sugar". "We will need to put the tooth to sleep" is recalled as "We will need to put you to sleep". Writing down key messages may decrease problems of interpretation.

"Childrenese" (choosing the right words)

The dental team needs to develop a specialised vocabulary to communicate with children. The manner in which information is presented to a child influences how they behave. Explain what is going to happen in simple, non-threatening language. "I am going to put this tooth to sleep so I can mend it for you" would be insulting to most adolescents but quite acceptable to a five- or six-year-old. Words like "injection", "needle", "jab" should be replaced by "freeze" "spray", etc. Some examples are given in Table 2-1 but many dental teams invent their own alternatives. A nine-year-old might

Table 2-1 **"Childrenese" terms for dental equipment**

Dental equipment	"Childrenese"
Slow handpiece	Buzzy bee
Air rotor	Whizzy brush or Mr Whistle
Triplespray/inhalation sedation	Magic wind
Local anaesthetic	Jungle juice or sleepy juice
Giving a local anaesthetic	Spray your teeth off to sleep
Rubber dam	Rubber raincoat
Rubber dam clamp	Clip or button
Fissure sealant	Tooth paint
Suction	Hoover
Amalgam	Silver star
Prophylaxis head	Tickling stick
Plaque	Bugs

Based on Fayle and Crawford, Making Dental Treatment Acceptable to Children (1997).

respond better to "force shield" (fissure sealant), "alien gunge" (plaque) and "Captains Fearless, Buzz and Careless".

It is also best to avoid a phrase like "There is nothing to worry about" or "This won't hurt at all", as they suggest that there may be something to worry about or that it might hurt. In other words, they achieve what you were trying to avoid!

Voice tone
Remember that the manner in which you say something is just as important as what you say. For young children, the tone of your voice is what they hear, and for many anxious patients a soft, reassuring voice that sounds calm has a better effect that a brusque businesslike voice saying the same words.

Key Points
- Enthusiasm may motivate.

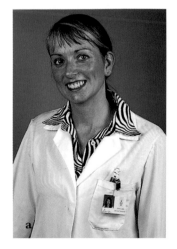 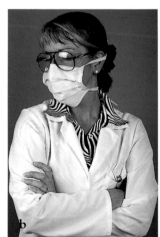

Fig 2-11 (a) Friendly dentist; (b) unfriendly dentist.

- Boredom spreads.
- Your patient's tone of voice may indicate if a message is being received or ignored.

Non-verbal Communication

Remember that communication is a two-way process: you are giving the patient as much information as they are giving you. This communication is often subconscious and may be far more accurate than the verbal messages that we give and receive. If you are not careful you may not give the message you intended. Some specific examples of non-verbal communication are given below (Fig 2-11).

Face
- Your face can add to or undermine your verbal message (disbelief, disapproval, dislike, surprise can be detected).
- Smiling is a powerful tool and has been shown to motivate.
- When you have a mask on you hide your face but a smile can be heard when you speak (Fig 2-12).

Eyes
- Eye contact establishes trust at the outset of an appointment.
- For best effect you must have the patient at the same level you are. (This can be a challenge with children.)

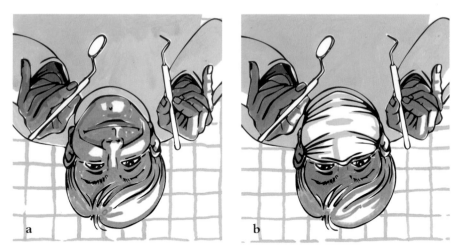

Fig 2-12 How children see us (a) unmasked; (b) masked.

Gestures and body posture
- Anxious patients fidget and fiddle more than relaxed patients.
- Crossing your arms as you talk may imply disapproval, especially if you also tap a foot!

Body contact
- A touch on the shoulder (in the presence of the parent and dental nurse) combined with a sympathetic tone may help reduce anxiety.
- Handshakes may increase confidence for some parents.

Appreciate that communication pathways are more complicated when young children are involved. The patient-dentist interaction that occurs with an adult patient is replaced by a three-way pathway between the child-parent-dentist. All three trying to communicate with each other may result in confusion rather that communication. Moreover, the dentist and parent can then send conflicting information to the child (see Chapter 4).

The Dental Environment (What Messages are You Sending?)

The dental surgery is an unfamiliar place to a many children, with strange smells and alien instruments. It has rules that are understood by the dental team and perhaps by the child's parents but which are still a mystery to the child. All these unknown things provoke anxiety in children. To overcome them, create an atmosphere in which a child feels comfortable and "safe" (Fig 2-13).

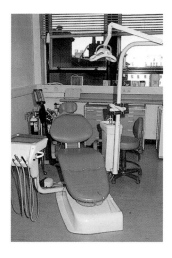

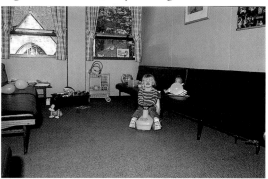

Fig 2-13 Even a well-designed modern surgery can look unwelcoming.

Fig 2-14 Child-friendly waiting room.

This can be achieved in a number of ways. It may be possible to use part of the waiting area to create a play zone for children, with activities to keep them occupied. Children who are sitting with nothing to do are far more likely to worry about what is going to happen or concentrate on other possibly anxious patients. Posters and pictures for children should be at the correct height for them and update everything periodically to ensure books and comics still look new and inviting and will appeal to a wide age range of both genders (Fig 2-14).

The co-ordinated effort of the whole dental team is also essential. Clear communication with the child and their family in an inviting atmosphere allows the unknown to become familiar in small steps. Ensuring that suitable intervals exist between appointments and leaving sufficient time within appointments helps the dentist to remain in control and plan treatment in appropriate stages.

Practical Tips

- Child communication has to be age specific.
- Get the environment right with
  - a "children's corner" in the waiting room, screened from anxious adults
  - "child-friendly" (primary) colours
  - children's books
  - toys

- posters positioned at child height
- pinboard for drawings of "going to the dentist"
- colouring sheets and badges
- puppets
- demonstrations of what to expect (for example, books about "going to the dentist").
- Train your staff to be friendly.
- Use age-specific language.
- Remember communication is more than just words.
- SMILE.
- Put the child at the centre.

Further Reading

Barker T. Patient motivation. In: Kidd EAM, Joyston-Bechal S. Essentials of Dental Caries. 2nd edn. Oxford: Oxford University Press, 1997.

Bernstein DA, Kleinknecht RA, Alexander LD. Antecedents of dental fear. J Pub Health Dent 1979;39:113-124.

Fayle S, Crawford PJM. Making dental treatment acceptable to children. Dent Profile. Sept 1997:18-22.

Freeman R. The case for mother in the surgery. Br Dent J 1999;186:610-613.

Geboy MJ, Muzzio TC, Stark AM. Communication and Behavior Management in Dentistry. Baltimore, MD: Williams and Wilkins, 1985.

Wright GZ, Alpern GD. Variables influencing children's cooperative behaviour at first dental visit. J Dent Child 1971;23:124-128.

Chapter 3
Child Taming II:
The Dental Team

Aim

This chapter aims to demonstrate how all members of the dental team can work together to manage children.

Outcome

Every individual team member should be able to participate actively in the delivery of dental care to each child who attends the practice, in a way that is both complementary to and supportive of his or her colleagues (Fig 3-1).

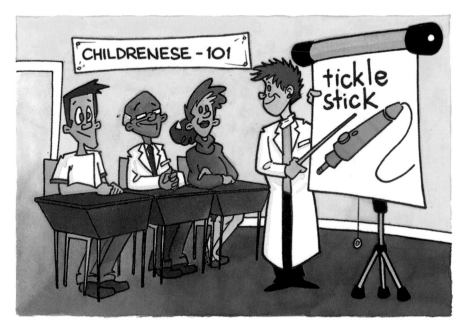

Fig 3-1 Team training.

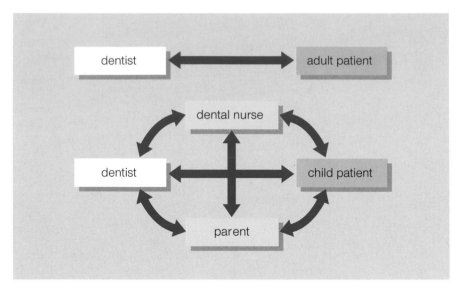

Fig 3-2 Lines of communication between adult patient and dentist is usually two-way. With children, communication lines can be more confusing.

Introduction

Each member of the dental team has a part to play in ensuring that a visit to the dentist is a pleasant experience. This means that dental surgeons have to decide how they want their practice to operate and each member of the team must understand what their role is and why it is important (Fig 3-2). Lines of communication with children can become very confusing unless ground rules are drawn from the outset.

Dental Team Roles

The Dental Receptionist
The receptionist has a key role since she or he is the first member of the dental team that the child meets (Fig 3-3). A professional, caring attitude on the telephone and when the parent arrives with the child helps to reduce parental anxiety and thus the anxiety of the child. The easiest way to do this is to SMILE (and as a smile can be heard in your voice when you speak, this works over the telephone too).

Sending a *Pre-appointment Letter* (see Appendix 1) prior to the first appointment can familiarise both child and parent with the practice and tells them

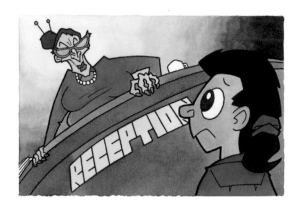

Fig 3-3 The face that greets.

what to expect during the first visit. The receptionist can confirm the contents of the letter with children who are coming to the practice for the first time as this is reassuring and helps establish their trust. Having appropriate toys and books can assist children by giving them a normal activity while they are waiting for their appointment and will help to take their mind off the forthcoming visit (Fig 3-4).

The child should be the centre of attention, so ensure your team uses the child's name to welcome them individually as well as addressing the accompanying adult. The receptionist must also assist the dentist by arranging suitable appointment times for anxious children since they will need a series of appointments at short intervals apart to allow the dentist to build on the progress of each visit. Each clinician needs to determine how often and long these appointments should be and guidelines should be available for all reception staff. Treating anxious children need not be time consuming; appointments can be kept short since many children find it difficult to concentrate or keep their mouth open for too long.

Practical tips for the receptionist.
- Keep your telephone voice friendly.
- SMILE.
- Welcome the child and know his or her name.
- Keep the waiting area "child friendly".
- Schedule appointments appropriately.

The Dental Nurse
The dental nurse and the dentist have to work together to manage the anx-

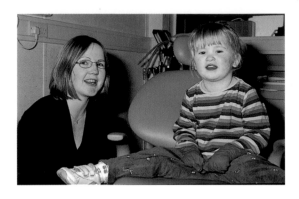

Fig 3-4 Get down to the child's level. Note the dental gloves!

ious child. The role of the dental nurse is to assist the clinician by anticipating his or her requirements and at the same time providing reassuring, calm support for the child. Get the surgery ready before the child enters so that he or she is neither alarmed nor distracted by the preparation of instruments and materials. If local anaesthesia is to be used, the syringe should be made up in advance and kept out of the child's view until it is required.

The dental nurse may have to keep the child entertained whilst the dentist is taking a history from the parent and this is a good opportunity to give the child "positive" information such as "It's fun to have your teeth polished".

Children can be easily overwhelmed and confused but this can be avoided if one person only addresses the child at a time, preferably from the child's height and using suitable language. Therefore, it is imperative that the dental nurse not only avoids distracting the child's attention from the dental surgeon (thus giving them a chance to build up a rapport with the child) but also tries not to use words such a "sharp", "hurt", "needle" and "drill". Once the dentist starts to interact with the child, they are the sole communicator and at this point the dental nurse usually remains quiet to help the child concentrate on one voice (Fig 3-5). The extent to which individual dental teams talk to patients will vary; what is essential is that the dental surgeon establishes how and when they wish the dental nurses to talk to children and when they wish to be the sole communicator. If parents or guardians are in the room they should understand their role too (see Chapter 4).

To avoid crowding around an anxious child, the dental nurse may have to help the dentist regulate the number of people in the surgery - by only inviting the child and one parent into the room at a time, for example. A polite suggestion, *"the surgery is small"* or *"the waiting room is more comfortable"* seldom causes offence to other accompanying relatives.

Practical tips for the dental nurse
- Prepare the surgery ahead of the visit.
- Smile and know the child's name.
- Talk to the child when the dentist needs the parent's attention.
- Use appropriate language.
- Regulate entry into the surgery.

The dentist (and colleagues)

The attitude of the dental operator towards the child is probably most significant in determining success or failure. Research has shown that every behaviour demonstrated by the dentist provokes a behavioural response from the child. In other words, the dentist can use his or her own behaviour to overcome or increase a child's anxiety response. Interestingly, studies comparing anxious and non-anxious patients have found that the anxious patient frequently refers to his or her dentist as cold, unfriendly or uncaring. In contrast, low-anxiety groups say that their dentists are gentle, caring or kind. This can also be extrapolated to include a dental hygienist or dental therapist.

One study looking at dentists' actions in response to fear-related behaviour in children found that immediate direction, specific reinforcement, asking how they felt and gentle pats or squeezes on the shoulder or hand resulted in a decrease in the young patients' anxiety levels and improved behaviour in the dental chair. Ignoring a child's feelings or verbal reassurance had no effect on their behaviour, while coercion, coaxing or put-downs actually made the children's behaviour worse.

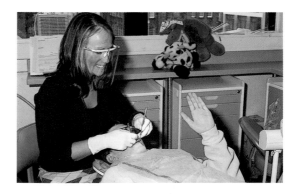

Fig 3-5 A "stop signal" gains trust.

Taken together, these findings suggest that the most effective action a dentist can show to gain a child's cooperation is empathy. Empathy is *the recognition of, or entering into the feelings of another person* and can be demonstrated by showing understanding and caring. Questioning about the child's subjective feelings by asking *"Why are you afraid ?"* and finding out specifically what the child is afraid of is often enough to start to gain the child's trust and cooperation. Other questions such as *"Are you OK?"* or *"Do you feel fine?"* during treatment puts an anxious child further at ease.

Counterproductive actions should be avoided. Constantly giving verbal reassurance - for example, "This wont hurt", makes the child consider the possibility that it may. Telling a patient "There is nothing to worry about" is a good way to make them worry; coaxing or bribing the child ("You can have a sticker if you are good") is also ineffective.

Practical tips for the dental operator
• SMILE.
• Show empathy.
• Ask about your patient's feelings.
• Reinforce good behaviour.
• Use gentle pats on the shoulder to maintain contact with the child.
• Avoid reassurance (it does not work and may make things worse).
• Do not coax or bribe (these do not work either).
• Take care not to belittle your patients: it may make them more anxious.

General Recommendations
• Put the child at the centre.
• Consider using pre-appointment letters.
• Clarify lines of communication.
• Ensure each member of the team uses the same language.
• Ensure that team members understand their individual roles.

Further Reading

Rosengarten M. The behavior of the pre-school child at the initial dental visit. J Dent Res 1961;40:673.

Weinstein P, Getz T, Ratener P, Domoto P. The effect of dentists' behaviors on fear-related behaviors in children. J Am Dent Assoc 1982;104:32-38.

Wright GZ, Alpern GD, Leake JL. The modifiability of maternal anxiety as it relates to children's cooperative dental behavior. J Dent Child 1973;40: 265-271.

Chapter 4
Parent Training

Aim

This chapter aims to review the importance of parents in providing dental treatment for children. Strategies to ensure a positive parental contribution will be outlined and issues surrounding the informed consent process will be discussed.

Outcome

On completing this chapter, the dental team should be able to develop a strategy to get the parent fully engaged in the delivery of oral health care and by so doing increase the likelihood of successful completion of treatment and of better life-long oral health (Fig 4-1).

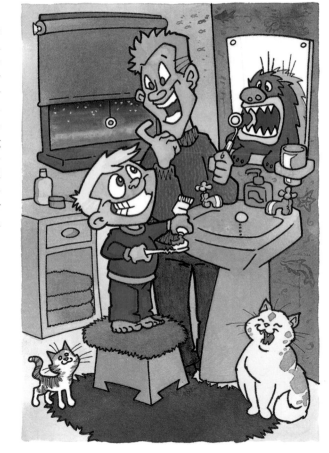

Fig 4-1 Parent training.

Introduction

The dental team, in a paediatric dentistry context, needs to be expanded to include the parent or guardian. One of the key aims of the oral care of children is to create a long-term interest in ongoing prevention and by so doing ensure improved dental health in the future. To achieve this the parents must be fully involved.

The treatment alliance

The dentist must establish a relationship based on trust with the child and with the accompanying adult to ensure compliance with preventive regimes and to allow treatment to occur. This "treatment alliance" is essential, as dentists rely on parents to bring the child in the first place and many aspects of preventive care can only be achieved when parents and the dental team work together (see below, Psychological Preparation). Indeed, a realistic treatment plan cannot be successfully formulated without the full involvement of the parent (Fig 4-2).

Many dentists have firm views on whether a parent should be present when dental treatment is carried out. However, parents also have views and many prefer to be there during treatment, especially if their child is young or attending an initial visit.

The major concern for dentists is the potential of the parent to disrupt treatment by inappropriate communication or by exhibiting anxiety themselves. The desire to exclude parents may also reflect the fact that many dentists are used to a one-to-one relationship with a patient and find the three-way interaction threatening. However, involving the parent in the planning stage and outlining their role as a passive but silent helper may provide a comforting presence without unhelpful interference.

Adverse parental effects
Dentists seek to exclude parents for a number of different reasons, including
- their potential to confuse communication by:
  - repeating what the dentist says (annoying both child and dentist)
  - intercepting the dentist's commands (acting as a barrier between dentist and child)
  - dividing the child's attention between parent and dentist
  - dividing the dentist's attention between child and parent

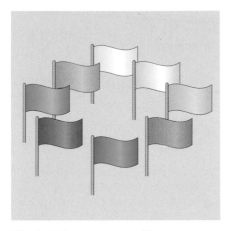

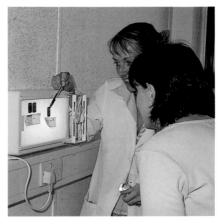

Fig 4-2 The treatment alliance.

Fig 4-3 Dentist and parent need to be "on the same side".

 – using inappropriate reassurance ("It won't hurt")
• behaviour contagion (transferring their own anxiety)
• well-intentioned but improper preparation
• discussing negative aspects of dental treatment within hearing of the child (reinforces vicarious learning)
• threatening the child with dental treatment ("The dentist will have to take your tooth out if you don't let her fill it!").

All of these can be avoided or overcome if the dental team take some time to explain the rules to the family (Fig 4-3).

Making parents part of the dental team
Research suggests that a child's behaviour once in the dental surgery is unaffected whether a parent is present or not. The exception to this is with very young children (under 4 years of age) who behave better with their mothers present. Separation anxiety is a normal developmental stage, and it has been shown to be a good indicator of dental anxiety in childhood. Thus, for very young children, a parental presence is important whereas for older children, a parental presence appears not to have such a clear effect on child behaviour but may be important to the parent. What is essential is that individual practitioners explain their practice policies regarding parental presence to parents.

Psychological preparation

Psychological preparation of an anxious child is best performed by the parent. However, the practitioner should offer guidance for this role, or the preparation may not have the desired effect. Such preparation is most effective when a systematic programme involving rehearsal and role-playing is used in the home. To be successful, the dentist not only has to motivate and involve the parent in the treatment but also to teach them how to prepare for each dental visit. This ensures that the parent knows what will happen at the next appointment and can ask questions in advance - thus avoiding questions at the start of the next visit when the dentist should be concentrating on the child.

Parental preparation
- Parents should use the same non-threatening vocabulary as the dental team ("childrenese"), such as "tickle", "sleepy juice" , "brush" and "spoon" instead of "hurt", "needle", "drill" and "excavator".
- Encourage parents to help the child practise in readiness for the next visit by "playing dentist". This is particularly effective when impressions are required: the child can be given an impression tray to take home to practise putting into the mouth. Alternatively, a disposable mirror can be used to examine a doll's teeth.
- Advise parents to hide their own dental anxiety, or have the child accompanied by an adult who is not anxious.
- Teach parents to use encouraging positive messages such as: "Its nice to have your teeth polished. I have mine done too".
- Teach parents to avoid using unhelpful reassurance that will raise anxiety such as: "The dentist won't hurt you" or "There is no need to worry".

Treatment planning and parental involvement

Treatment planning should not be carried out without involving both parent and child, although clearly the balance of responsibility will change as the child ages. Many elements of care rely on the parent, particularly for young children. Food choices, control of snacking and oral hygiene are usually under parental control (although responsibility for brushing teeth is often delegated to the child at too early an age). We have also outlined above the role of the parent in psychological preparation.

Every treatment plan requiring intervention should have a preventive component and once the examination is complete the dentist and parent need to meet to discuss the treatment that is planned. This should include

Preventive treatment
- The parent's role in terms of controlling access to sugary foods and drinks, completing dietary analysis records and assisting with toothbrushing.
- The dentist's role, such as monitoring, fissure sealants, etc.

Restorative treatment
- The parent's role in terms of attending for appointments and preparing the child.
- The dentist's role including the need for local anaesthetics, the number of teeth to be treated, an estimate of the number of visits, etc.

Surgery rules
- Whether the parent can be with the child for appointments or not.
- These need to be clear to the parent regarding the role you wish them to play if they are allowed to be present in the surgery (Table 4-1).

Are you talking to the right person?

Because of consent issues, it is important to know to whom you are talking. But be sure that the person you are talking to is responsible for carrying out the task you are discussing - for example, toothbrushing or buying treats.

Table 4-1 **Sharing dental care with a parent**

Dental role	Parental role
Explain the surgery rules	Accept the role assigned
Teach psychological preparation	Prepare child for visits
Explain treatment plan	Accept commitment to attend
Explain need for diet analysis	Complete diet analysis
Provide diet guidelines	Control access to sugar
Demonstrate toothbrushing	Comply with toothbrushing regime
Discuss use of fluorides	Control fluoride toothpaste
Encourage and support family	Continue to follow guidance
Monitor fissure sealants	Attend for check-ups
Provide good restorative care	Attend for treatment
Explain the parent's role	Prepare the child for visits

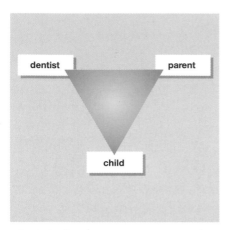

Fig 4-4 The communication triangle.

Discussion of the treatment plan should be used to identify the number of visits required, the type of treatment to be undertaken and the parent's concerns regarding the treatment. For example, if you are planning to introduce local anaesthetic at the next visit you should try to ensure that questions and worries are dealt with today, not during the appointment next time. Children have short attention spans and over-long descriptions of the procedure about to be carried out, for the parent's benefit, may be distressing for the child who is waiting for you to start. Finally, the discussion gives you an opportunity to outline any preparation you require the parent to undertake prior to the next visit (Fig 4–4).

Case conferences

A case conference will save on time later. Use it to inform the parent of the dental needs of the child. This develops their understanding of the necessity for operative intervention, the role of preventive care and, as such, gets the parent "on board". A visit-by-visit management strategy can then be planned, giving due regard to the emotional level and likely capability of the child to cope with the planned treatment. If conscious sedation is to be employed, the need for this and the proposed technique should also be discussed. At all times, appropriate language must be used together with an explanation of alternative methods of pain and anxiety control.

The child and their parent should be given an opportunity to ask for further information about any aspect of the proposed treatment and questions should be answered truthfully and in good faith.

For a successful case conference
- Talk the parent through the clinical needs of the child.
- Speak in positive terms - for example, "together we can fix this by ...".
- Remember that you are all working in a collaborative effort to solve the child's dental problems.
- Avoid jargon.
- Use language at a level that everyone can understand.

- Consider avoiding explicit fear-provoking detail when the child is listening.
- Give the parent and the child an opportunity to participate in the decision-making process.
- Make sure everyone is clear that they have an individual role/responsibility in the successful completion of the treatment.
- Build in some thinking time if required (another parent or guardian may need to be consulted).
- Give the parent and child information sheets as appropriate - for

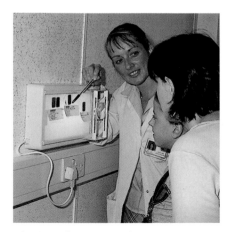

Fig 4-5 The case conference.

example, describing the sedation technique. This both aids retention and prevents distortion of the key facts (Fig 4-5).

Consent

When dealing with adults, consent is frequently assumed by the patient's willingness to sit in the chair and allow treatment to take place ("implied consent"). With children, consent cannot be inferred in this way. The parent or legal guardian needs to consent to treatment on the child's behalf. It is essential that the clinician knows who the accompanying adult is and confirms that they are able to give consent on the child's behalf. Only a parent or legal guardian can do this (Fig 4-6).

While a child under 16 years of age might be considered "competent" to consent themselves, it is still advisable to obtain parental/guardian consent whenever possible. How-

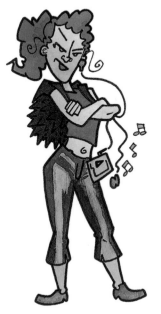

Fig 4-6 A competent child ...?

35

ever, within this framework the dentist should always try to respect the wishes of the child when obtaining consent. Indeed, for more mature children and especially adolescents, this kind of involvement in their dental care is an essential requirement for successful treatment completion. Furthermore, a child who is unwilling or incapable of cooperation is often not suitable for treatment as a degree of compliance is required if success is to be assured. It follows therefore that, irrespective of age, children should voluntarily accept treatment and should not be coerced in any way to accept treatment against their wishes.

Practical Tips

- Know who the accompanying adult is.
- Always treat preschool children with a parent present (this prevents separation anxiety).
- Teach parents how to prepare themselves and their children.
- Discuss the treatment plan with the parents.
- Be sure that parents understand their role in their child's care ("We are all on the same side").
- Remember to ensure you always have valid informed consent.

Further Reading

Frankl SH, Shiere FR, Fogels HR. Should the parent remain within the dental operatory? J Dent Child 1962;29:150-163.

Hawley BP, McCorkle AD, Witteman JK, et al. The first dental visit for children from low socio-economic families. J Dent Child 1974;41:376-381.

Wright G, Starkey PE, Gardener DE, Curzon MEJ. Child Management in Dentistry. Bristol: Wright, 1987.

Wright GZ, Alpern GD, Leake JL. A cross-validation of the variables affecting children's cooperative behaviour. J Can Dent Assoc 1973;39:268-273.

Chapter 5
Behavioural Management Techniques

Aim

The aim of this chapter is to present the common behavioural management techniques that the dental team can use to deliver care successfully to children (Fig 5-1).

Outcome

On completing this chapter you should be able to undertake, either alone or in combination, a number of behavioural management strategies and identify which are the most suitable for individual patients.

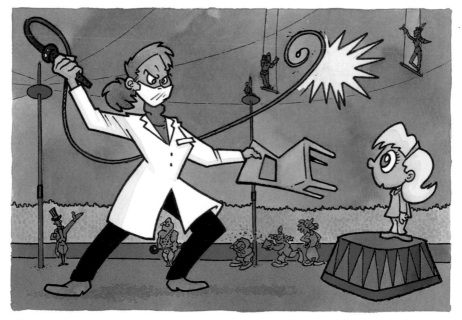

Fig 5-1 Use behavioural management to tame children!

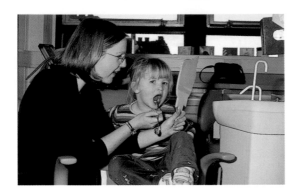

Fig 5-2 A happy and memorable first visit to the dentist.

Introduction

The label "uncooperative" is frequently applied to a child who behaves poorly in the dental surgery. Occasionally the term is used after his or her first visit. The term implies that a child is deliberately being awkward, but this is not usually true. Their behaviour normally reflects how they are feeling. We need to remember that, unlike adults, a child has no choice when attending the dentist: a grown-up brings them. Children have relatively limited communication skills and are less able to express their fears and anxieties verbally. When a child cannot cope, they attempts to "escape" and the change in behaviour that you see in the dental chair is often a child who is anxious or uncomfortable and has no other way to cope or inform you of their difficulty. Behaviour-management strategies try to help children accept the various feelings and experiences associated with dental treatment.

Behavioural Management

Graeme Wright (1975) defined behavioural management as "the means by which the dental health team effectively and efficiently performs treatment for a child". He suggests that a "positive dental attitude" is the aim of behavioural management. More recently he has refined the definition so as not to imply just behaviour necessary to complete a given task, but to include creating a long-term interest on the patient's part for ongoing prevention and for future improved dental health. To do this the dentist must establish relationships based on trust with the child and accompanying adult to ensure compliance with preventive regimes and allow treatment to occur (the "treatment alliance") (Fig 5-2).

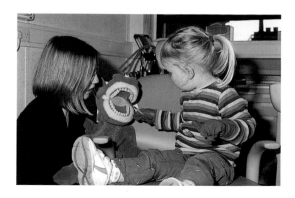

Fig 5-3 Acclimatisation.

- Behavioural management methods are about communication and education.
- The relationship between a child, the child's family and the dental team is a dynamic process that is the key to success.
- Behavioural management starts before the patient arrives in the surgery and employs dialogue, voice tone, facial expression and touch.
- No single method will be applicable in all situations. Instead, the appropriate management technique(s) should be chosen based on the individual child's requirements.

Behavioural management techniques

"Tell–Show–Do"

"Tell-Show-Do" is a technique used widely to familiarise a patient with a new procedure. It employs concepts from learning theory and has been adopted by many paediatric dentists. The technique works well combined with behaviour shaping and is well accepted by parents, although there is little research relating to its use. It appears to be most valuable with low-anxiety levels: there is no evidence to support its usefulness with very anxious children. More recently it has been shown to reduce anticipatory anxiety in new child patients, although it was less useful in children with previous negative dental experiences (Fig 5-3).

The *tell* phase involves an age-appropriate explanation of the procedure. The *show* phase is used to demonstrate the procedure - for example, demonstrating with a slow handpiece on a finger. The *do* phase is initiated with minimum delay - in this case a polish. The language used must be appropriate to the child's age - many dentists use a personal version of this "childrenese"

(Table 2-1) and the whole dental team must adopt the same approach. Specifically emotive or negative words are avoided.

Behaviour-shaping and positive reinforcement

Many dental procedures require quite complex behaviours and actions from our patients. Adults have learnt that they come into the dental surgery, lie down and have their teeth examined. They understand that they need to be quiet and to allow the dentist to look at their teeth. A child patient does not know what is expected of them and the dental team needs to teach them how to behave. For children this requires small, clear steps. This process is termed "behaviour shaping". It consists of a defined series of steps towards ideal behaviour. This is most easily achieved by selective reinforcement.

Reinforcement is the strengthening of a pattern of behaviour, increasing the probability of that behaviour being displayed again in the future. Anything that the child finds pleasant or gratifying can act as positive reinforcement. Stickers or badges are often used at the end of a successful appointment. However, the most powerful reinforcements are social stimuli - such as, facial expression, positive voice modulation, verbal praise and approval through hugging. A child-centred, empathic response giving constant feedback and specific praise (for example, "I like the way you keep your mouth open") has been shown to be more effective than a general comment such as "Good girl." As with "Tell-Show-Do", the use of age-specific language is imperative.

Positive Reinforcement

Children want to please you and respond well to encouragement and praise - for example, "That's great, when you open wide like that I can see really well", or "Well done, it really helps when you sit so still like that". Research has shown that "drip-feeding" positive encouragement throughout the appointment is a good way to train a child to become an ideal patient. For best effect, positive reinforcement, like praise, needs to be given throughout the session immediately after appropriate behaviour is demonstrated. Praise at the end alone does not seem to work: you must make it clear to the child which behaviour is being rewarded.

There is also good evidence that ignoring inappropriate behaviour and rewarding good behaviour tends to extinguish the former. In contrast, commenting on it is more likely to result in it occurring again, as the child has received the desired result: your attention! For example, the child who asks "How long until you finish?" is likely to keep repeating the question if you stop and answer the first time. It is usually better to ignore the question and find something positive to comment on.

"Tell-Show-Do", behaviour shaping and positive reinforcement in action

Many dentists use these techniques all the time without realising it. The techniques might be used together to allow a first examination.

Dentist: OK, I've shown you how the chair works. Now I'd like to look in your mouth and count your teeth. Pop your head on the pillow for me.

[Child lies back on pillow]

Dentist: That's great, are you comfortable?

[Child nods head]

Dentist: Let's have a look in your mouth. How wide you can open you open?

[Child opens mouth a little]

Dentist: That's good, but I can't see your back teeth. See if you can open wide enough for me to see them.

[Child opens mouth wider]

Dentist: Wow, that's really wide. That makes it a lot easier to see your teeth. [To dental nurse, Susan] If I fall in, Susan, will you pull me out? Have a little rest then I am going to count your teeth. Close your mouth.

[Child closes mouth]

Dentist: OK, this time I'm going to count your teeth using this little mirror. Can you see how small it is? It's just the right size to count your teeth. All right, are you ready? Let's see if you can open again.

[Child opens mouth wide again]

Dentist: That's really good. You are opening your mouth really well and that helps me a lot. [Begins counting]

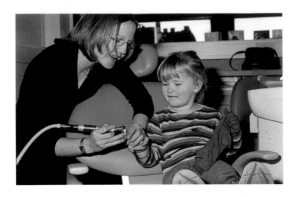

Fig 5-4 "Tell-Show-Do".

The process has been broken down into small steps and the child is taken through each stage. Adding them together ("behaviour shaping"), the dentist is continuously praising the child as he or she follows each step ("positive reinforcement"). At the same time, the explanation tells the child what is going to happen, rehearses it, and then carries it out ("Tell-Show-Do"). The same process can be used for any procedure (Fig 5-4).

Enhancing control

A major cause of anxiety is feeling out of control. Therefore, if an anxious child is allowed to feel that they have some degree of control, anxiety is alleviated. The patient can be given a degree of control over your behaviour through the use of a "stop signal". Such signals have been shown to reduce pain during routine dental treatment and during an injection. The stop signal, usually raising an arm, should be rehearsed and you must respond quickly when it is used, as failing to do so will increase anxiety instead. Children may overuse the signal until they learn to trust you, and it is essential to accept that they are learning to control their anxiety and to trust you. If you fail to honour the agreement their trust is lost.

It is also possible to use a signal to proceed. Here the patient indicates that they are ready for you to carry on. This process engages the child in the visit. They are no longer passive recipients of your care; rather, they may actively control you by stopping you and/or allowing you to proceed (Fig 5-5).

Distraction

This approach aims to shift the patient's attention from the dental setting to some other situation, or from a potentially unpleasant procedure to something else. Cartoon films have been shown to reduce disruptive behaviour

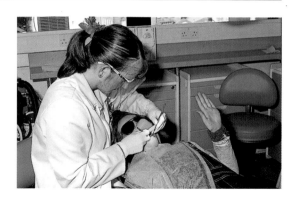

Fig 5-5 A "stop signal" can even be used during conscious sedation.

in children when combined with reinforcement (where a child knows the video will be switched off if they do not behave). Playing music or telling the patient stories can work just as well: there is evidence that audiotapes may be even more effective.

Short-term distractions, such as diverting attention by pulling the lip as a local anaesthetic is given or having patients raise their legs to stop them gagging during radiography, may also be useful. The dentist who talks while applying topical paste and administering local anaesthetic is also using distraction with words.

In addition, allowing a child to watch some part of a procedure with a hand mirror further reassures them and involves them more closely in their dental treatment. During lengthier procedures older anxious children might be encouraged to bring along a personal stereo to listen to as a demonstration of the dentist's trust and understanding.

Systematic Desensitisation
This technique helps individuals overcome specific fears or phobias through repeated contacts. A hierarchy of fear-producing stimuli is constructed, and the patient is exposed to them in an ordered manner, starting with the stimulus posing the lowest threat. In dental terms, fears are usually related to a specific procedure such as use of local anaesthetic. First, the patient is taught to relax (this is essential because it is not possible for a person to feel both relaxed and anxious at the same time). The best-known technique uses progressive relaxation of muscle groups starting with the feet and working up the body.

Once the patient has learned how to relax they are exposed to each stimulus in the hierarchy in turn, only progressing to the next when they feel able to do so. An example of a hierarchy for local anaesthetic is shown in Table 5-1. For true phobias, several relaxation sessions with a psychologist or dentist who has received training in relaxation or hypnosis techniques may be required. Indeed, one reported case required nine hour-long sessions with a therapist. However, a similar approach can be used for children who have had a negative experience in the past.

Table 5-1 Systematic desensitisation hierarchy for phobia related to dental local analgesic injections

1. Instructions on muscle relaxation and or relaxation breathing
2. Explanation of components of local anaesthetic equipment
3. Look at an assembled dental syringe
4. Explanation and demonstration of effect of topical anaesthetic
5. Information and facts about local anaesthetic administration
6. Hold an assembled dental syringe on the palm of the patient's hand
7. Hold an assembled dental syringe by the patient's face
8. Hold an assembled dental syringe inside the patient's mouth
9. Hold an assembled dental syringe (needle guard removed) on the palm of the hand
10. Hold a syringe (guard removed) by the side of the face
11. Hold the syringe inside the mouth (guard removed)
12. Replace the guard and hold the end of the syringe against the mucosa overlying the injection site
13. Press the syringe (guard in place) over the injection site
14. Place topical anaesthetic
15. Remove the guard and hold the syringe inside the mouth
16. Place the needle in contact with the mucosa over the injection site.
17. Place the needle in contact with the mucosa and insert some pressure
18. Hold the needle in contact with the mucosa and inserting enough pressure for the needle to penetrate the mucosa
19. As in 14, but deliver a minute amount of local analgesic solution
20. As in 14 but deliver a normal amount of local analgesic solution

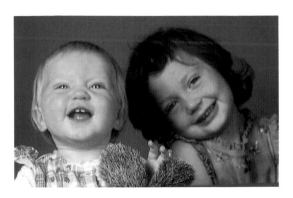

Fig 5-6 This pre-schoolchild will emulate her older sister's behaviour in the surgery .

Modelling

The modelling technique is based on the psychological principle that people learn about their environment by observing others' behaviour, using an actor, either live or on video, to exhibit appropriate behaviour in the dental environment. This demonstration of appropriate behaviour via a third party will help decrease anxiety by showing a positive outcome to a procedure the child requires themself, and illustrates the reward for performing well. For best effects, the actor should be a similar age to the target child, should exhibit appropriate behaviour and be praised. They should also be shown entering and leaving the surgery (Fig 5-6).

Watching an older and more confident child undergoing treatment has been shown to be a positive influence. Often the presence of an older sibling in the dental surgery will improve the behaviour of a younger child. This can be attributed to the younger child's attempt to emulate and win the approval of an older brother or sister. This technique can be used to greatest effect in children between three and five years of age and is particularly useful for their first visit to a dentist.

Key Points

- The aim of behavioural management is to instil a lifelong positive attitude to dental health.
- Behavioural management is a dynamic process between the dental team, the child and their parent, so make sure everyone in the surgery knows what their role is during treatment.
- Get the family involved by explaining what will happen at the next visit and have them help prepare the child.

- Facial expression, voice tone, body language and touch are all critical elements of child management (remember that the tone of your voice is often of more consequence than what you say). You can distract and sooth if you talk to your patients as you treat them.
- "Tell–Show–Do" can be used for all patients, but remember to make the language appropriate for each child.
- Try to break dental treatment into small manageable steps for each patient, and explain as you go along.
- Remember that children like to please you, so tell them when they do. But be specific or the child does not know what they did well!
- Involve your patients in their own treatment by giving them a degree of control over *you*.
- Let your patients know you care. Talk to them. Ask if they are all right.
- Remember to smile. It shows in your eyes and can be heard in your voice.

Further Reading

Addleston HK. Child patient training. Chicago Dent Soc Fortnightly Rev 1959;38:7-9, 27-29.

Fayle S, Crawford PJM. Making dental treatment acceptable to children. Dental Profile 1997;Sept:18-22.

Fields, HW Jr, Machen JB, Murphy MG. Acceptability of various management techniques relative to types of dental treatment. Pediatric Dentistry 1984;6:199-203.

Weinstein P, Nathan J The challenge of fearful and phobic children. In: Dental phobias and anxiety. Dental Clinics of North America 1988.

Chapter 6
Sequential Treatment Planning

Aim

The aim of this chapter is to demonstrate how a sequential treatment plan can be built to facilitate successful child management.

Outcome

Having read this chapter the practitioner should be able to adopt a step-by-step approach to treatment planning for operative procedures in children irrespective of their initial presenting level of cooperation (Fig 6-1).

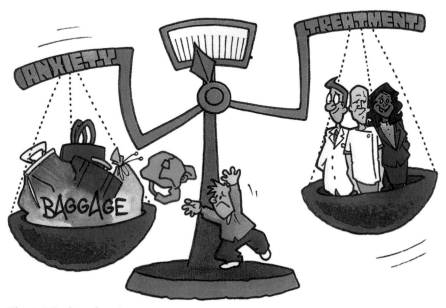

Fig 6-1 Scales of anxiety.

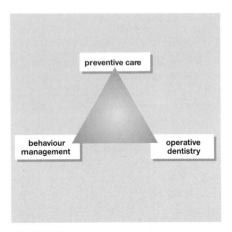

Fig 6-2 Behavioural management, preventive care and operative dentistry are interwoven.

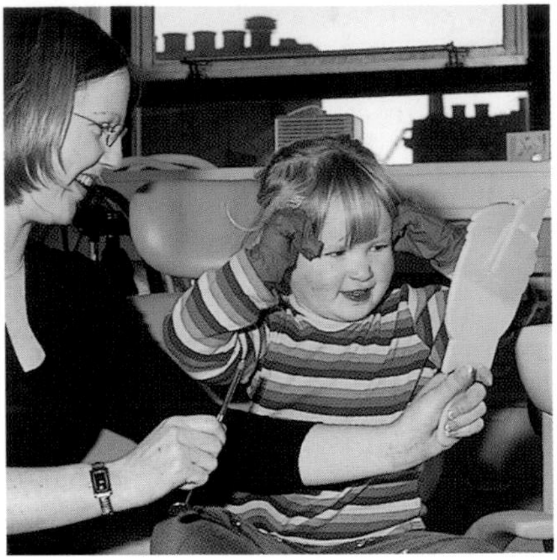

Fig 6-3 Dentist and child acclimatising.

Introduction

Previous chapters have shown that emotional maturity, previous dental experience and the influence of the family, the dental surgery environment and the dental team all affect child management. Behavioural management techniques have been reviewed and in subsequent chapters we will explore the use of conscious sedation. At this stage it is appropriate to demonstrate how non-pharmacological and pharmacological techniques can be woven together in a sequential treatment plan (Fig 6-2).

Gradual Introduction of Instruments and Procedures

Hill and O'Mullane (1976) show that 60% of anxious children can be helped by sequential treatment planning in which dental instruments and procedures are introduced gradually. This has to be carried out in a prearranged manner and therefore involves forward planning. It need not be time consuming. A typical treatment plan that could be used to treat an anxious child is shown in Table 6-1(a). It shows that some items of treatment can be completed while other instruments and procedures are being introduced (Fig 6-3).

Acclimatisation is about taking a child with no dental experience and assisting them to become ready to accept dental care. It is a combination of techniques ("Tell-Show-Do", behaviour shaping, positive reinforcement and

48

Table 6-1 **Sequential treatment planning**

	(a) Behavioural management	(b) How to add inhalation sedation
Visit 1	• Simple oral examination • Discuss diet • Invite child to bring tooth brush next visit • Take radiograph home to practise with	• Show inhalation sedation equipment on leaving • Let child help to assemble it ("Are you good at LEGO?")
Visit 2	• Brush the child's teeth using his or her own toothbrush • Invite the child to sit in the chair • Take radiographs • Introduce "Mr Buzzy brush" at slow speed by polishing the teeth • Blow the teeth dry with the 3:1 ("wind")	• Introduce and briefly use inhalation sedation using oxygen only with child standing, just before they leave (they will happily try this, especially in the knowledge that their treatment is already finished for this visit) • Parent-dentist conference and signed consent. • Give parent the information leaflet
Visit 3	• Apply fissure sealant and/or temporary dressings in stages • Introduce saliva ejector ("sucky-straw")	• Use inhalation sedation
Visit 4	• Remove carious tooth tissue with a hand excavator • Introduce slow-speed drill ("bumpy brush") • Perform small buccal and cervical restorations	• Let child position the nosepiece for themselves
Visit 5		• Continue to use inhalation sedation

Items 1(a) and 2(a) can often be combined in the first visit

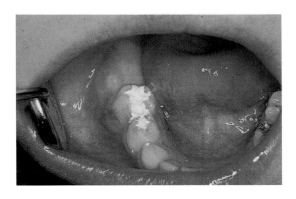

Fig 6-4 Stabilisation can be effective in securing future cooperation.

psychological planning), integrating these, with conscious sedation if required, into the operative plan.

Stabilisation/Temporisation

Leaving active caries untreated is never appropriate. Converting an active open cavity into a quiescent inactive cavity is (Fig 6-4). The active caries can be treated without local anaesthesia, with minimal tooth tissue removal, as part of a holistic approach to the management of a "pre-cooperative" or anxious child. Even when there is no attempt to render the cavity caries free, dressing with a fluoride leaching-agent may buy time by slowing the progress of disease and thereby prevent pain and sepsis, whilst facilitating coping through acclimatisation. However, it is essential that the parent knows that this is just a temporary measure to reduce the bacterial load and to slow caries progression whilst the child is undergoing behavioural management and receiving preventive care. This can be a part of the dentist-parent conference.

Pragmatic treatment planning

The cornerstone of restorative dentistry is preventive care. After all, restorations placed in a mouth still undergoing active decay rapidly fail and soon need replacing. This is not only disappointing for the dental team but also leaves the family questioning why they were placed in the first place. The child feels the treatment has failed them (Fig 6-5).

"Grey" areas
In an ideal world one would hope that all children would have the "best care possible". But what is best care? Do we mean high-quality restorative care?

50

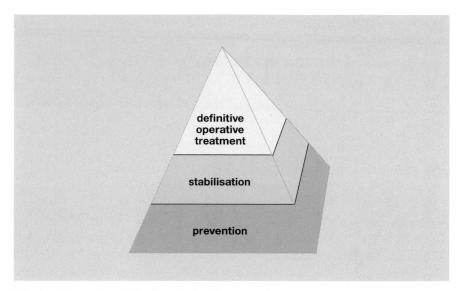

Fig 6-5 Prevention is the foundation for operative care.

If we do, should it be achieved irrespective of the child's ability to cope and the parents' desire to receive (or attend for) this? This is simply not possible for every child presenting with dental caries at every time-point in their lives. A "pre-cooperative" child may need general anaesthesia to achieve this at further cost and increased risk. Indeed, a child may be potentially treatable to this high standard under local anaesthesia but not necessarily at the point in time that they present. For example, if they have had a bad day at school or a recent disruption in their family life, prolonged operative treatment may be impracticable. In situations such as these, stabilisation may be the initial treatment of choice rather than immediate, perfect quadrant dentistry.

Neither the child nor the dental team gains in a struggle to complete a plan that was simply inappropriate in the first place. A systematic approach is required to assess each child and their family well enough to tailor the treatment plan to fit both the child's dental needs and the family's capability to accept the treatment. This cannot be done adequately at the introductory visit. However, acclimatisation and prevention can be implemented while this assessment process is progressing. Professionals complementary to dentistry, such as dental hygienists and dental therapists, can be particularly valuable in this initial stage.

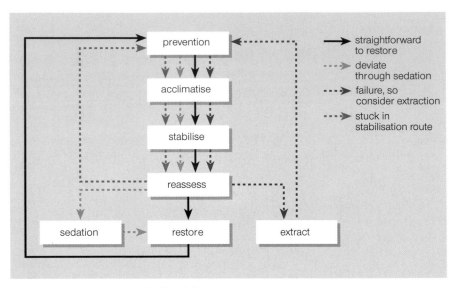

Fig 6-6 The prevention feedback loop.

Clinical Scenario

We will use the example of a four-year-old child and his mother attending for his first visit because of occasional toothache. He is healthy and brushes his own teeth. Examination reveals

- interproximal caries affecting upper incisor teeth
- occlusal cavities into dentine on upper first molars
- mesial cavities on lower first molars.

At this point you cannot tell how he will respond to care and it is possible to outline a number of possible approaches. Some are represented diagrammatically in Fig 6-6. The first phase for all of these options includes prevention, acclimatisation and stabilisation. A possible strategy is outlined in Table 6-2.

Reassessment

Following stabilisation, stop and review the progress of both the child in the surgery and the family's preventive practices to determine what happens next.

1. If the child has accepted treatment so far and the family is responding to

Table 6-2 **Preventive protocol**

Prevention	Acclimatisation	Stabilisation
First Visit • Disclose plaque and give toothbrushing instruction • Give diet advice in relation to both sugar and acid frequency • Give instruction on how to complete the diet diary and ask patient to bring the completed diary next visit • Fluoride	• Introduce the use of a "hand signal" to the patient • Ensure that the teenage patient understands that they have a role/share in their dental treatment: that we are partners in their care (hence the reason for asking them to complete a "patient contract") • Demonstrate mixing of cement dressing • Demonstrate the slow-speed hand-piece, polishing cup and polishing paste and introduce by polishing the patient's fingernail • Polish teeth, invite the patient to use the hand signal if required • Be empathetic: ask "Are you OK"; "Are you coping"; "Does it taste OK?" • Discuss the patient contract and ask patient to sign it • Prepare the patient for the second visit	• Dress (reversible pulpitis only, i.e. vital pulp) asymptomatic carious cavities with glass ionomer cement • Introduce hand instruments • Disc interproximal cavities in primary incisors
Second Visit • Assess plaque control and reinforce tooth-brushing instructions • Check diet diary and repeat/reinforce diet advice • Apply fluoride varnish to teeth and also to previous dressings (to recharge them)	• Remind patient about the "hand signal" • Polish teeth again, invite the patient to use the hand signal if required	• Dress any remaining (reversible pulpitis only, i.e. vital pulp) asymptomatic carious cavities with glass ionomer cement • Disc any remaining anterior interproximal cavities

preventive protocols, introduce local anaesthesia and continue with restorative care in subsequent visits.

- Describe, then use, the topical anaesthetic gel.
- Describe its "bubblegum" smell and flavour.
- Explain that it makes "everything it touches go numb".
- Allow child to smell the gel.
- Give child a hand mirror.

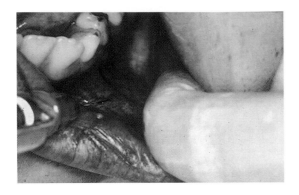

Fig 6-7 Pain-free dentistry is important.

- Place some topical gel on a cotton wool roll and direct child to put the gel onto the lower lip.
- After two minutes let child *gently* place a probe on the bottom lip to compare "pinchiness" and hence understand the positive effect of the gel in relation to administration of a local anaesthetic.
2. The child has coped with stabilisation but needs a lot of support. Home care is improving and the family are keen. Consider using some sedation to assist with the introduction of local anaesthesia and restorative care.
3. The child has coped with stabilisation (albeit with some problems) but most treatment has been on the parent's lap. The family is assisting with prevention but the child is not ready for operative treatment more at this stage. Wait. Maybe the child's ability to cope will improve. In the meantime, reinforce the preventive advice, show the family the dressings and explain that they need to be checked regularly.
4. The child has struggled with acclimatisation and stabilisation and there has been no improvement over two or three visits. Prevention has not improved and there are episodes of spontaneous pain. Consider extracting the teeth.

Other options

In other words, children presenting with similar clinical problems may receive very different treatment plans. The first option is perhaps the most straightforward for the dental team. It assumes a cooperative patient and a family complying with preventive regimes with a minimum of six visits before they enter the preventive/recall loop. The fourth option is the least desirable to most dental teams. However, it allows preventive input, removes the imme-

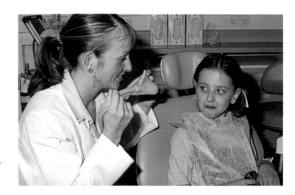

Fig 6-8 Introducing the child to sedation is a part of the acclimatisation therapy.

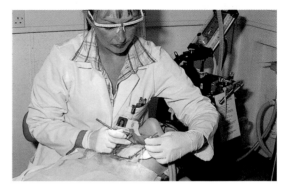

Fig 6-9 Good sequential planning results in quality operative dentistry.

diate cause of pain and potential sepsis, and provides the possibility of treatment-free recall visits if the family returns for ongoing care (Fig 6-7).

Treatment Planning with Local Anaesthesia and Inhalation Sedation

The concept of sedation is to reduce fear, anxiety and stress and to promote a feeling of comfort and well-being. Clearly, pain control is a fundamental part of this and so the acceptance of local anaesthesia is also often incorporated into the planned dental procedure (Figs 6-8 and 6-9).

For optimal effect, nitrous oxide inhalation sedation has to be introduced to the anxious child from the beginning of treatment. Table 6-1(b) demonstrates how inhalation sedation can be incorporated into a treatment plan.

55

Practical Tips

- Definitive restorative treatment depends on a solid prevention and management foundation.
- The child's stage of development and level of anxiety must be taken into account when treatment planning.
- The treatment plan must be tailored to fit the child.
- Stabilisation of caries coupled with prevention may be a launch pad for definitive restorative care once cooperation improves.

Further Reading

Hill FJ, O'Mullane DM. A preventive programme for the dental management of frightened children. J Dent Child 1976;Sept–Oct:326-330.

Chapter 7
Conscious Sedation1: What It is and When to Use It

Aim

The aim of this chapter is to:
- define conscious sedation
- position paediatric dental sedation in the United Kingdom in relation to other parts of the world and to medicine
- present the relevant child anatomy and physiology in relation to paediatric dental sedation
- outline the risks, benefits and complications of paediatric conscious sedation
- explore when to use conscious sedation.

Outcome

The information in this chapter should enable dental practitioners to determine when sedation is appropriate for the management of an anxious child.

Introduction

In previous chapters various options for successfully managing children in dental practice have been presented. But for some children conscious sedation may be needed to augment an existing behavioural management strategy. The dental team should not forget, however, that behavioural management strategies continue to underpin the delivery of dental treatment under conscious sedation. So in paediatric dentistry, sedation must always be combined with behavioural management - integrated and tailored to meet not only the needs of each child, but also each planned procedure (Fig 7-1).

Conscious sedation for children is different from conscious sedation for adults. A child's anatomy and physiology differ from an adult's, which means that the way they react to sedative drugs is also different. Adult studies cannot be applied to children just as paediatric studies cannot be extrapolated for use in adults. Moreover, whilst there is a huge research evidence base supporting paediatric dental sedation, this has mainly been reported by specialist paediatric dentists outside the United Kingdom.

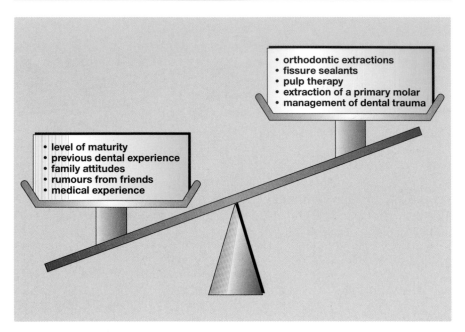

orthodontic extractions
- fissure sealants
- pulp therapy
- extraction of a primary molar
- management of dental trauma

- level of maturity
- previous dental experience
- family attitudes
- rumours from friends
- medical experience

Fig 7-1 Anxiety baggage.

What Sedation is Not

Remember that conscious sedation adds to conventional behavioural management techniques it does not replace them, as sedative drugs alone cannot replace good communication or create the right environment in which the child feels safe. Moreover, like all other treatment provided for children, conscious sedation must not be separated from an acknowledgement of each individual child's level of emotional and intellectual maturity. In short, conscious sedation for children is not a "quick fix". Instead, it is a part of the armamentarium that dentists use to help children accept dental treatment.

So What is Conscious Sedation for Dentistry?

Different definitions of dental sedation may be found in the literature, for example:
> "A state of depression of the central nervous system enabling treatment to be carried out, but during which verbal contact with the patient is maintained throughout the period of sedation."

"The administration of an agent prior to dental treatment for the purpose of obtaining an alteration of the patient's psychic response and subsequent relief of apprehension and anxiety."

"A minimally depressed level of consciousness that retains the patient's ability to maintain a patent airway independently and continuously, and respond appropriately to physical stimulation and/or verbal command ... the drugs and techniques used should carry a margin of safety wide enough to render unintended loss of consciousness unlikely."

While the definitions vary, the underlying theme is clear: sedation is the use of agents to decrease anxiety levels while maintaining a responsive patient. Within the United Kingdom the contemporary guidance must be followed and all suggested practice within this text complies with the current General Dental Council (GDC) recommendations for conscious sedation. The current GDC definition of conscious sedation is as follows:

"A technique in which the use of a drug or drugs produces a state of depression of the central nervous system enabling treatment to be carried out, but during which verbal contact with the patient is maintained throughout the period of sedation. The drugs and techniques used to provide conscious sedation for dental treatment should carry a margin of safety wide enough to render unintended loss of consciousness unlikely. The level of sedation must be such that the patient remains conscious, retains protective reflexes, and is able to understand and to respond to verbal commands."

A World-Wide View of Paediatric Dental Sedation Literature

There has been extensive research into sedative drugs and drug combinations throughout the world with oral, intravenous, rectal and inhalational routes being reported. Given this variation, it is often difficult to discover whether or not the sedative level achieved matches the contemporary definition of conscious sedation. Indeed, in many cases it is clear that the reported regimen is unlikely to comply.

A prime example of this is "deep sedation", which has been defined as "a controlled state of depressed consciousness or unconsciousness from which the patient is not easily aroused, which may be accompanied by a partial or complete loss of protective reflexes, including the ability to maintain a patent airway independently and respond purposefully to physical stimulation or verbal command."

Thus the deep sedation practised, for example, in North America, chiefly by paediatric dentistry specialists, is considered in the United Kingdom to be general anaesthesia and, as such, the operating dentist is required not only to have a qualified anaesthetist present to administer the sedation but also be sited on or near an acute hospital.

United Kingdom Culture and Practice

Cultural differences exist between nations, and these set limits on the way dentists manage anxious or uncooperative children. In the United Kingdom, dentistry and general anaesthesia have close historical links that may partly explain why general anaesthesia is used far more for dental extractions in children compared with most other countries. On the other hand, the papoose board, a restraining device most commonly used in North America to facilitate dental treatment, is less acceptable to British parents for the same purpose. Similar reservations exist about some forms of sedation for dental treatment, especially in a primary care environment. For example, rectal sedation, which is successfully used in several countries and has a good evidence base to support its use, is unpopular with United Kingdom parents and therefore not usually employed.

Therefore, one of the difficulties in interpreting literature from different sources is determining its applicability to United Kingdom practice. This includes how acceptable the technique will be to the United Kingdom population and whether or not it complies with GDC guidelines. In other words, the fact that a study demonstrates that a particular regimen is successfully used in children abroad does not mean that that the same protocol can be used in the United Kingdom. Things that are unlikely to be acceptable to most United Kingdom practitioners and parents include:
- combinations of drugs
- child restraints (papoose board)
- mouth props.

Moreover, where combinations of techniques are employed it is hard to determine how much of the success is due to the sedative regime and how much to the management techniques used. Not surprisingly, some of these deep sedation and restraining techniques also raise questions concerning informed parental consent, professional acceptance and the possibility of litigation (Fig 7-2).

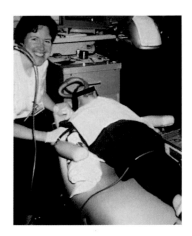

Fig 7-2 Sedation in other parts of the world may not meet UK standard of conscious sedation (MTH in the USA).

Sedation in Medicine

It is unwise to attempt to crowbar sedative regimens from medicine into dentistry. The level of sedation required for dentistry is quite different from other medical fields - for example, the child has to stay perfectly still for radiography but has to be conscious enough to keep his or her own mouth open for dentistry. Moreover, even the technique is different. A prime example of this is the use of Entonox nitrous oxide in maternity units. In dentistry, nitrous oxide inhalation sedation involves the titration of nitrous oxide with oxygen to achieve the desired effect, whereas the Entonox in maternity units delivers a fixed 50:50 concentration of nitrous oxide to oxygen. As such, the two techniques bear little resemblance to each other and the safeguards built into the dedicated dental machine are absent. For this reason only dedicated dental inhalation machines should be used.

Crash Course in Child Anatomy and Physiology

Airway anatomy
- Large head, short neck, large tongue.
- Narrow nasal passages.
- Nasal breathers at birth.
- High anterior larynx.
- Larynx narrowest at cricoid cartilage.
- Large floppy epiglottis.

Respiratory physiology
- Low functional residual capacity (FRC).
- Closing volume is greater than FRC up to 5 years of age, leading to increased ventilation/perfusion (V/Q) mismatch.
- Horizontal ribs, weak intercostals muscles leading to relatively fixed tidal volume.
- Oxygen consumption is high (6ml/kg/min compared to 3ml/kg/min in adults).

Temperature regulation
- High surface-area-to-body-weight ratio.
- Large head-surface-area and heat loss.
- Require a higher temperature for a thermoneutral environment.
- Immature responses to hypothermia (poor shivering and vasoconstriction).
- Brown fat metabolism which increases oxygen consumption.

Nervous system
- Increased incidence of periodic breathing and apnoeas.
- Ventilatory response to CO_2 is more readily depressed by opiates.
- Immature neuromuscular junction leads to increased sensitivity to muscle relaxants.

These differences in paediatric anatomy and physiology mean that a child can become hypoxic more easily than an adult.

Complications during Paediatric Conscious Sedation

The main complication related to paediatric conscious sedation is hypoxia. Other complications are
- nausea
- vomiting
- inadvertent general anaesthesia (over-sedation)
- staff addiction/drug abuse.

Benefits of Conscious Sedation

- Promotes patient welfare and safety.
- Facilitates the provision of quality care.
- Minimises the extremes of disruptive behaviour.
- Promotes a positive psychological response to treatment.

Don't Forget Local Anaesthetic (Analgesia) is a Drug Too

In situations where local anaesthetic is also necessary, remember that it, too, is a pharmacological agent. The result of this is that when even a single sedative agent is added, at least two drugs, the sedative and the local anaesthetic, will have been administered to the child. Clearly, the planned treatment must take the therapeutic safety of local anaesthetic into account and so the provision of operative dentistry under conscious sedation is sometimes limited, by virtue of the dose of local anaesthetic, to one or two quadrants. As such, full-mouth care in one visit under general anaesthetic almost always translates into multiple visits once a conscious sedative technique is adopted as an alternative.

Local anaesthesia: maximium dosage
Lignocaine 4.4mg/kg
2.2ml cartridge of 2% solution contains 44mg of the active agent.
For a 3- to 5-year-old (wt 20kg) 2 cartridges.

Prilocaine 6mg/kg
3% solution contains 30mg/ml.
For a 3- to 5-year-old (wt 20kg) 1.75 cartridges (approx.).

When to Use Sedation

Some children may already be anxious about receiving treatment; others may simply not be ready to cope with the amount of treatment that they require. Hill and O'Mullane report that 60% of children offered behavioural management coupled with sequential treatment planning manage to accept dental treatment. Nevertheless, this implies that the remaining 40% will need either sedation or, indeed, general anaesthesia. The difficulty for the dentist drawing up the treatment plan is determining into which category an individual patient falls (Fig 7-3).

In this section we will focus on the key reasons for using sedation:
• reducing the child's level of anxiety
• using sedation to prevent anxiety.

Assessing the level of anxiety
Despite acknowledging that anxiety in children is prevalent, dentists regularly embark on courses of treatment without first assessing anxiety level. Wouldn't it be great if there was a simple ready-reckoner that dentists could

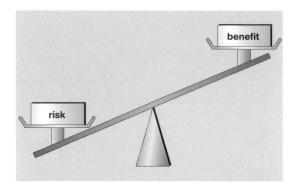

Fig 7-3 Risk-benefit balance.

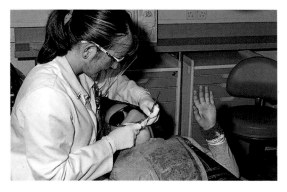

Fig 7-4 The dentist-patient relationship is the key to success.

use to assess the level of anxiety and, by doing so, assist in the choice of the best management tool? Sadly, it isn't that simple. We have demonstrated previously that assessment of the level of a child's anxiety is based on a number of factors: the stage of emotional development, individual character, previous medical and dental experiences (the child's own and the experiences of his or her family and peers) together with how well the dental team has succeeded in providing a safe, friendly environment (Fig 7-4).

Recognising and assessing anxiety
There are three ways to assess anxiety:
• physiological assessment
• behavioural observation
• self-report methods.

Physiological assessment is useful for research purposes as it measures heart rate or other parameters – so-called objective data. However, such techniques are rarely useful in the surgery. Behavioural observation relies on the patient's actual behaviour in the surgery being rated by the operator or trained observer(s) using standardised scales. These may be useful in child patients who may find questionnaires difficult. However, the expression of anxiety changes as we age. Children usually manifest anxiety overtly as they have not yet learned how to hide their emotions and are more likely to display their fears.

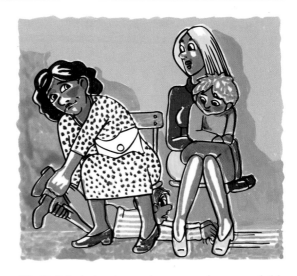

Fig 7-5 Sedation is not the answer for every child.

As a consequence, dentists can spend much more time trying to manage children, and behavioural management techniques are well recognised as methods to assist both the child and the dentist.

Most adults and many older children have learned to alter their behaviour to conform to socially acceptable patterns and are more likely to suffer in silence. They may not overtly manifest their anxieties, and may not appear to be anxious in the surgery. As a result the reassurance they require is often withheld. Interestingly, anxiety is often at its greatest in the waiting room, where clinicians are least likely to observe it. Fidgeting, pacing, sitting on the edge of the chair, repetitive limb movement or startled reactions to noise may be manifested by the anxious adult while waiting for the appointment. One study observed patients' behaviours in the waiting room and in the dental surgery but also used self-report questionnaires for the patients and dentists. Adults reporting high anxiety by questionnaire behaved differently in the waiting room where they felt free to display signs of their anxiety but behaved the same as the low-anxiety group in the dental surgery. The correlation between the dentist and patient rating of anxiety was low. In other words, dentists do not always identify anxious patients (Fig 7-5).

Self-report questionnaires have been used for many years. The dental anxiety scale (DAS) developed by Corah is one of the most widely researched and has been modified by some researchers to include a question on local anaesthesia (the modified dental anxiety scale – MDAS). This originally asked four questions about how patients would feel in various situations, such as having a dental visit tomorrow, or waiting while the dentist gets the drill. It then gives five possible answers ranging from relaxed to physically ill, with a maximum score of 20: the higher the score, the more anxious the patient. The modified scale includes a fifth question about local anaesthesia (Table 7-1).

Used correctly, these questionnaires can give an approximate measure of a patient's dental anxiety and an indication of specific concerns. However, they are not widely used. One recent survey of 328 United Kingdom dental practitioners listed in the British Society for Behavioural Sciences Directory revealed that only 20% of those asked used anxiety questionnaires with adult patients and 17% of them with child patients.

Table 7-1 **Asking the parent about their child using the modified dental anxiety scale (MDAS)**

	Not at all	Slightly	Fairly	Very	Extremely
1. If you went to your dentist for treatment tomorrow, how anxious would you feel?					
2. If you were sitting in the waiting room (waiting for your turn to see the dentist), how anxious would you feel?					
3. If you were about to have a tooth drilled, how anxious would you feel?					
4. If you were about to have your teeth scaled and polished, how anxious would you feel?					
5. If you were about to have a local anaesthetic injection in your gum, above an upper back tooth, how anxious would you feel?					

"Preventive" sedation

Sometimes conscious sedation must be used on children who don't appear anxious to prevent anxiety developing following a potentially traumatic operative procedure (Fig 7-6).

A typical example of the preventive use of conscious sedation is the low-caries-risk, regular attender who needs orthodontic extractions. Another example might be when a child who has previously had only a dental examination or simple operative procedure (fissure sealants, for example) needs restorative treatment or extractions for the first time - especially when the treatment planned, using local anaesthesia for the first time, is in more than one quadrant.

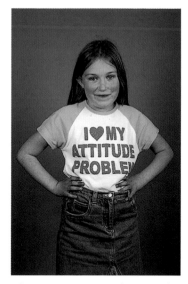

Fig 7-6 Even a regular attender may find some treatment too much for them.

The bond of trust that has developed between the child and dentist over time might be strong enough to permit one extraction or restoration under local anaesthetic or, indeed, one primary molar pulp therapy. However, next time around, this trust may be overstretched. Whilst some children, in a supportive dental environment, might still allow the dentist to complete the subsequent operative procedure, their attitude towards dentistry in the future is at risk of irrevocable damage. Indeed, there is evidence to suggest that children who receive the most treatment are most likely to develop anxiety.

> Ideally, the use of conscious sedation, particularly nitrous oxide inhalation sedation, should be considered for immediate implementation <u>before</u> the first planned procedure takes place, to avoid later anxiety.

Second time around

You may not be the first dentist to see a patient. Where a child has had a previous unpleasant dental experience and is anxious because of this, conscious sedation can be used to help them. In this case sedation is used to overcome dental anxiety not to prevent it occurring in the first place.

Key Points

- Paediatric anatomy and physiology mean that a child can become hypoxic more easily than an adult.
- Hypoxia is the major complication in the sedation of paediatric dental patients.
- Conscious sedation is not a substitute for behavioural management.
- Conscious sedation is not a "quick fix".
- Studies from other countries and from other medical specialities may not be appropriate for use by dentists in the United Kingdom.

Practical Tips

- Always remember to calculate the dose of local anaesthetic, especially when sedative drugs are to be added.
- Integrate conscious sedation with behavioural management techniques in the sequential treatment plan.
- The assessment of a child's level of anxiety may help to alert the dental team to manage anxiety (Table 7-2).
- Tailor management strategy to fit the needs of each individual child.
- Introduce conscious sedation early, especially when treatment is likely to be difficult or lengthy, to prevent anxiety occurring.

Table 7-2 Example of a visual analogue scale to use with children

Put a <u>mark on the line</u> below to show us how you feel <u>now</u>.

_____

NOT AFRAID AT ALL   VERY AFRAID

Put a <u>mark on the line</u> below to show us how you usually feel about going to the dentist.

_____

NOT AFRAID AT ALL   VERY AFRAID

Further Reading

Corah NL. Assessment of a dental anxiety scale. J Dent Res 1969;43:596.

Cote CJ, Karl HW, Notterman DA, Weinberg JA , McCloskey C. Adverse sedation events in pediatrics: analysis of medications used for sedation. Pediatrics 2000;106:633–644.

Cote CJ, Notterman DA, Karl HW, Weinberg JA , McCloskey C. Adverse sedation events in pediatrics: a critical incident analysis of contributing factors [see comments]. Pediatrics 2000;105:805–814.

Dailey YM, Humphris GM, Lennon M. The use of dental anxiety questionnaires: a survey of a group of UK dental practitioners. Br Dent J 2001;190:450–453.

Humphris GM, Morrison T, Lindsay SJE. The modified dental anxiety scale: United Kingdom norms and evidence for validity. Comm Dent Health 1995;12:143–150.

Meechan JG. Practical Dental Local Anaesthesia. London: Quintessence, 2002.

Selbst SM. Adverse sedation events in pediatrics: a critical incident analysis of contributing factors [letter, comment]. Pediatrics 2000 ;105:864–865.

Chapter 8
Conscious Sedation 2:
Preparing the Parent and Child

Aim

The aim of this chapter is to demonstrate how to prepare both the child and his or her parent for conscious sedation.

Outcomes

After reading this chapter the practitioner will
- be able to select those children who are most likely to accept treatment using sedation, particularly inhalation sedation
- confidently assess the child's dental needs
- recognise the role of good communication to ensure a successful outcome through parent and child participation
- obtain informed consent
- give appropriate pre- and postoperative instructions.

Introduction

The preparation of parent and child for conscious sedation is much more complex than a novice dental sedation team might at first have envisaged. However, time spent in this preparation will help make successful operative dental treatment under conscious sedation a reality for the anxious child and their family. The step-wise preparation outlined in this chapter also guarantees compliance with contemporary guidance in respect of safe sedation practice. Good preparation helps to avoid failed sedation visits, through better patient selection and parent engagement, and so saves time in the long run (Fig 8-1). These preparatory steps can be incorporated into the sequential treatment plan outlined in Chapter 6.

Preparing the parent and child includes
- Assessing the dental needs of the child.
- Assessing the medical health of the child.
- Assessing the potential cooperation of the child.
- The dentist parent child conference.

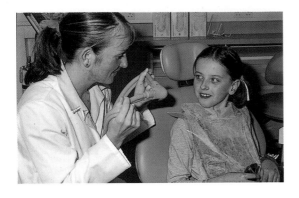

Fig 8-1 Preparing the child for conscious sedation.

- Gaining informed consent.
- Psychological preparation of the child.
- Fasting instructions, where relevant.
- Parental instructions prior to sedation visit.
- Compiling appropriate records.

Assessing the dental needs of the child

A full dental history and examination are essential parts of the assessment prior to sedation. Of particular importance is the dental and medical history as it is necessary to identify anxiety-provoking stimuli. This enables them to be avoided, where possible, and helps to tailor the dental management to limit the child's anxiety where it cannot. Once a specific stimulus is identified their likely reaction to that stimulus can be anticipated in advance of treatment.

Common anxiety-provoking stimuli in children are fear of the unknown and lack of control. Some children may remember unpleasant medical procedures - for example, giving blood samples or a recent school vaccination. There is also evidence to suggest that previous general anaesthetic extractions may cause dental anxiety. Some children associate "the mask" with their dental fear, so identify this if nitrous oxide inhalation sedation (IS) is being considered. Its introduction in such cases must include an assurance that it is "not like being put to sleep": a different thing entirely (Fig 8-2).

A complete and accurate diagnosis of a child's dental disease is also essential. In the case of dental caries both enamel and dentinal lesions need to be identified. Only 40% of dental caries is diagnosed clinically, so a radiographic

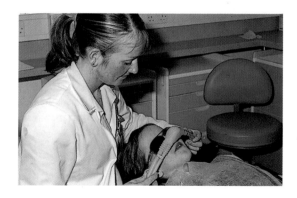

Fig 8-2 Introducing the nasal mask.

examination is essential accurately to treatment plan appropriate preventive and restorative care. The child must feel that he or she has completed treatment as they will lose confidence in the dentist should further treatment be required at every future recall. This can easily happen if enamel lesions are not identified and preventive therapy instituted. A holistic approach to the dental care of the child has to be adopted whilst the treatment plan is determined. This should include a caries risk assessment, sequential treatment planning, when to introduce local anaesthesia and how to interleaf prevention into the overall plan.

Assessing the Medical Health of the Child

We have already learned in Chapter 7 that the anatomy and physiology of a child differs from those of an adult and how easily children can become hypoxic. A full and up-to-date medical history is always relevant to every aspect of the practice of dentistry but there are some specific areas that need to be explored in greater detail whenever conscious sedation is considered. Dentists must ensure that a parent or guardian who is fully conversant with the child's health provides the medical history. Indeed, the complete assessment may have to be postponed if another close relative - for example, grandparent or aunt - has accompanied the child.

The medical history must include:
- cardiac defect, murmurs
- drug allergy
- respiratory diseases, including recent colds
- bleeding disorders
- immune compromising conditions

- previous problems with general anaesthesia or sedation
- a history of family problems with general anaesthesia or sedation
- current medication
- any other involvement with another dental or medical specialist.

Fitness for conscious sedation, or general anaesthesia

Fitness for conscious sedation, or general anaesthesia, is usually described in relation to the American Society of Anesthesiologists (ASA) Classification (Table 8-1). Generally, patients who can be categorised as ASA I and ASA II can be considered for conscious sedation in a primary care environment. Patients whose ASA categorisation is beyond this should be referred to specialist centres.

American Society of Anesthesiologists Classification

Within the ASA classification mild systemic disease refers to disease that does not affect the patient's lifestyle (hay fever or eczema, for example). Moderate systemic disease, in contrast, is disease that limits activity but is not incapacitating (for example, asthma that limits exercise).

In a dental clinic there are no facilities to investigate underlying medical disorders or to provide rapid support in the event of problems. For these reason only patients who are fit and well or who have mild medical conditions that do not affect their lifestyle should be treated outside of hospital. Only patients rated ASA I and 2 should be treated in primary dental care. General anaesthesia should be used with caution on ASA 3 and ASA 4 status patients, for whom it would be advisable to administer sedation in a hospital environment supported by an anaesthetist.

Table 8-1 **American Society of Anesthesiologists (ASA) classification**

Class I	A normally healthy patient
Class II	A patient with mild systemic disease
Class III	A patient with severe systemic disease
Class IV	A patient with severe systemic disease that is a constant threat to life
Class V	A moribund patient who is not expected to survive without an operation

When to be cautious

There are a number of factors where caution is required when sedation is considered:

- infants
- renal impairment
- hepatic impairment
- severe respiratory disease
- gastro-oesophageal reflux
- children already receiving opioids or other sedatives
- children receiving other drugs that potentiate the sedative duration (for example, macrolide antibiotics potentiate midazolam)
- children with cardiovascular instability or impaired cardiac function
- bleomycin therapy when nitrous oxide inhalation sedation is considered.

Rates of morbidity and mortality increase with extremes of age and with worsening ASA classification. In addition to this, drug metabolism may be affected in patients with renal and hepatic problems, so lower dosages of sedative agents may be required. Remember that all sedative drugs depress respiration. Therefore, children who already have impaired respiratory function due either to a pre-existing medical condition or to existing medication with other respiratory depressants have a greater risk of developing a reduction in circulating oxygen levels (hypoxaemia). The same is also true of those with deficient cardiac function. Nausea and vomiting are complications of sedation and the risk of gastric content entering the lungs increases in children with gastro-oesophageal reflux.

Assessing Cooperation

A degree of cooperation is required for most sedation techniques and so it is essential that the child must have some understanding of what sedation entails. There are no absolute age limits but "pre-cooperative" children may not be able to cope with some forms of sedation. A prime example of this is nitrous oxide inhalation sedation where the child has to agree to collaborate by breathing through the nosepiece. Similarly, a lack of understanding or willingness to collaborate might also hinder the success of conscious sedation for some children with learning disabilities. In this latter case, in particular, expert specialist advice might

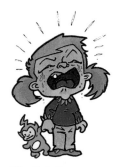

Fig 8-3 Pre-cooperative child.

be required, together with an anaesthetist to assist with the sedation during the dental procedure. Sometimes the option of general anaesthesia should be considered instead (Fig 8-3).

The Case Conference

Following completion of the dental and medical assessment the dentist must conduct a case conference with the parent and child. The parent of an anxious child is generally anxious too, particularly when they discover that their child needs operative dental treatment. Time set aside to explain to the child and parent together is important (see Chapter 4).

The case conference:
- helps develop the dentist–child relationship
- ameliorates the anxiety of the parent
- assists in the informed consent process
- saves wasted time later.

Involving the parent and child

The essential value of forming a bond between dentist and child together with the supportive role of the parent has been elaborated in previous chapters. When conscious sedation is being considered it is even more important to involve these key players. The necessity for conscious sedation together with the need for operative intervention and the role of preventive care need to be demonstrated. This facilitates the development of a visit-by-visit plan that can also take into account the emotional level and likely capability of the child to cope with the envisaged treatment. An explanation of the sedation technique proposed must then be discussed with both parent and child, using appropriate language. An explanation of alternative methods of pain and anxiety control can also be discussed at this point. The child and their parent should be given an opportunity to ask for further information about any aspect of the proposed treatment and these should be answered truthfully and in good faith (Fig 8-4).

The "sedation" case conference
- Remember that you are all working in a collaborative effort to solve the child's dental problems.
- Avoid jargon; use language at a level that everyone can understand.
- Explain the sedative technique proposed.
- Make sure everyone is clear that they have an individual role/responsibility in the successful completion of the treatment.

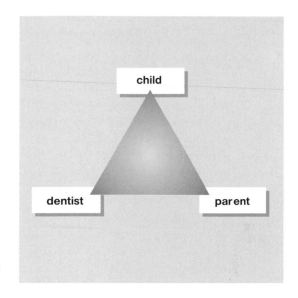

Fig 8-4 Interrelationships during sedation.

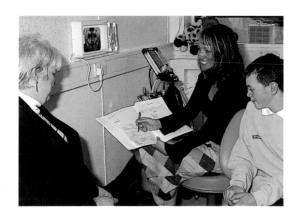

Fig 8-5 The case conference is a vital component of the consent process.

- Build in some thinking time, if required (another parent or guardian may need to be consulted).
- Give the parent and child information sheets describing the sedation technique.
- Give the parent and child the pre- and post- operative instructions (Fig 8-5).

Gaining Informed Consent

> "Consent is the voluntary and continuing permission of a patient to receive a particular treatment. It must be based upon adequate knowledge of the purpose, nature and likely effects and risks of that treatment, including the likelihood of its success and any alternatives to it."
> The Society for the Advancement of Anaesthesia in Dentistry (SAAD)

Like almost all aspects of dental care, consent is about communication. For children under 16 years of age it is usually necessary for a parent to consent. For consent to be valid, the parent, or a *competent* child, must be able fully to comprehend the information that has been provided and the treatment plan that has been discussed. Moreover, he or she has to assimilate this information before making a decision (Fig 8-6).

Informed consent for sedation must be obtained in writing and a copy attached to the patient record.

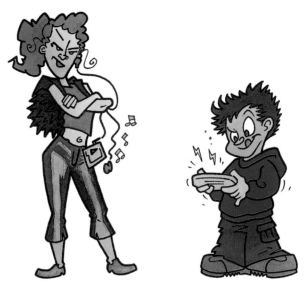

Fig 8-6 Who is competent to give consent?

Information that is Required before Sedation

- Child and parent must be given clear and comprehensive pre- and post-operative instructions in writing.
- Informed consent must be obtained in writing.
- Remind the parent or guardian that the child must have an adult escort.
- Advise the accompanying adult to bring no other children with them to the visit.
- Check that there is adequate arrangements for travelling home after the conscious sedation visit.
- Remind the parent or guardian to take care - for example, crossing roads.
- With the exception of nitrous oxide inhalation sedation, the child should remain home that evening and kept under supervision.

Psychological Preparation

Psychological preparation prior to the sedation visit is invaluable. When this support is also maintained during the procedure there is a positive additional effect to the relaxation and well-being of the child. Explanations about the proposed procedure have to be delivered by means appropriate to each individual child's stage of emotional and cognitive development. Positive reinforcement is valuable together with other more specific techniques such as guided imagery and play therapy. Indeed, play therapists have been shown to reduce the need for sedation. Psychological preparation, in addition to decreasing a child's stress, has also been shown to reduce parental stress.

Children who received a combination of systematic preparation, rehearsal and supportive care prior to each stressful procedure are less upset and give better cooperation, whilst their parents report significantly greater satisfaction and less anxiety compared with those who received a single preparation session or inconsistent support.

Psychological preparation includes (Fig 8-7):
- play therapy
- play acting to rehearse a procedure
- using relaxation to introduce new events
- using age appropriate language
- using tone and body language.

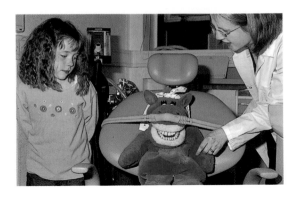

Fig 8-7 Rehearsal and play have a role in psychological preparation.

Fasting

There is a potential that food or liquid in the stomach could present an aspiration risk if patients become unconscious. The definitions of sedation and the techniques recommended in this text should ensure a wide margin of safety to prevent loss of consciousness. The need for fasting within this definition of conscious sedation, using drugs with wide safety margins, is still relatively controversial. Most anaesthetists would agree that it is sensible to limit the risk of gastric contents from entering the lungs further by implementing clear fasting regimes for all sedative agents with the exception of nitrous oxide inhalation sedation.

Recommended fasting regime for nitrous oxide
Where nitrous oxide is the only sedative used no fasting is required.

Recommended fasting regime for all sedatives except nitrous oxide
Prior to sedation the patient should have ingested:
- no solids for 6 hours
- no milk for 4 hour
- no clear fluids for 2 hours.

Parental Instructions Prior to Sedation Visit

In addition to specific advice on psychological preparation and fasting a number of other instructions must be given to the parent or guardian who is consenting to treatment. Whilst these are relatively simple they are best given as a written information sheet. An example is given in Appendix 2.

Compiling Appropriate Records

As with all other aspects of dental care, it is essential to maintain accurate dental records.

Before sedation the clinical record should record:
- a list of the anxiety-provoking stimuli
- a summary of the dental history and of the treatment required
- the reason why conscious sedation is needed
- evidence of consent
- written medical and anaesthetic/sedation history
- confirmation that the pre- and postoperative instructions have been given.

Following sedation the clinical record should record:
- written details of treatment undertaken
- written details of sedation used and the patient's reaction to it
- confirmation that the postoperative instructions have been given.

Practical Tips

- Take a thorough medical history and check for existing conditions and medication.
- Don't forget that sedation augments other behavioural management techniques but does not replace them.
- Conscious sedation needs to be part of a sequential treatment plan.
- Preparation of the child and parent will save time and ensure success.
- Informed consent and giving pre- and postoperative instructions can form part of the parent-dentist conference.
- Written pre- and postoperative instructions avoid parents having to remember essential details.

Chapter 9

Conscious Sedation 3: Preparing the Dental Team and Facilities

Aim

The aim of this chapter is to outline how the dental team and the surgery facilities need to be prepared before offering conscious sedation to a child.

Outcome

The dental practitioner should be able to
- develop the roles to be preformed by each member of the dental sedation team
- understand the appropriateness of both clinical and electronic monitoring
- handle all drugs safely, particularly nitrous oxide gas.

Introduction

Dental practitioners who wish to offer a conscious sedation service to their patients have a responsibility to ensure that they and their staff are appropriately trained to deliver best-quality care and to assist should a rare emergency arise. In Chapter 3 the individual, yet complementary, roles that each team member performs were presented. Whenever conscious sedation is offered to patients these roles are expanded further and it is even more important for the team both to be fully conversant with their own individual role and also to have the ability to transfer and integrate their skills to ensure the continued well-being of their sedated child patient. In addition to this, special consideration has to be given to the facilities and equipment in the dental practice where sedation is offered and to the continued health and safety of the dental staff.

Preparing the Dental Team

Each member of the dental team has a specific role to play in managing an anxious child and their escort when they present for the conscious sedation appointment. The key roles are:

- to prepare the dental team to manage both an anxious child and a sedated child
- to prepare the equipment.

Training

Before sedating a child, all members of the dental team must receive
- theoretical training
- practical training
- clinical training
- training in how to manage complications.

Each aspect of this training process must include the use of the specific sedative agent that has been planned for the child patient. It is also essential that the team has experience in the behavioural management of children and is competent in the operative procedures that are planned. Clinical and theoretical training in the provision of conscious sedation is not enough; the team must also be trained to recognise and to manage sedation-related complications. The ability to rescue the child is essential in the event of complications. Indeed, in a review of clinical incidents relating to sedation in children it was the inability to recognise complications and then subsequently rescue the child that lead to clinical incidents.

Every dental team already knows that there are specific guidelines in respect of training in basic life support to which they must conform, even if sedation is not being offered in the practice. Clearly, a team that offers conscious sedation to anxious children has to prepare further to ensure that that knowledge is retained and skills updated. To achieve this each member needs to be involved in a programme of continuous education and assessment relating to both operative paediatric dentistry and conscious sedation. Organisations that offer this kind of post graduate training in sedation are listed at the end of this chapter.

The receptionist

The receptionist is the face of the dental team and must be aware that the first contact can do much to alleviate or to cause anxiety as well as inspiring confidence in the success of the procedure. The role of the receptionist has been discussed already (Chapter 3) but there are some specific additional duties relating to conscious sedation that can be assumed by reception staff.

The receptionist has the pivotal role in the emergency protocol. They must be the person in charge of contacting the emergency services should this be required.

Key Roles and Duties

Dental receptionist

- Being the face of the dental team.
- Issuing pre-appointment letter.
- Ensuring pre-operative instructions are given and clearly understood.
- Logging appointment.
- Preventing crowding in the surgery.
- Confirming that the child has an appropriate escort and transport home.
- Completing anxiety questionnaires (if desired).
- Having a specific assignment in the event of an emergency.
- Updating knowledge of the emergency trolley inventory.
- Knowing basic life support.
- Implementing the emergency services protocol and facilitating patient transfer (if necessary).

Dental nurse

The dental nurse is a key member of the dental team in the management of the anxious child. Calm support and participation in behavioural management techniques are essential for any treatment to succeed. Do not underestimate the role of the dental nurse as a chaperone. Sadly, nowadays, every dentist, irrespective of gender, needs to be chaperoned for their own safety, but never more so when sedative drugs are used, as many sedative drugs cause hallucinations.

> THE DENTIST MUST BE CHAPERONED.

In conscious sedation for dentistry, the dental nurse often also acts as the sedation assistant by monitoring the sedated child and/or sedation equipment. Like the receptionist, he or she has specific assignments in the event of an emergency. The whole team should periodically practise these emergency scenarios. The dental nurse must have knowledge of the emergency trolley inventory and may also have the additional responsibility of ensuring that drugs are kept within their "use-by-dates". Finally, they should, like the rest of the dental team, be able to demonstrate basic life support skills.

Key Roles and Duties

Dental nurse
- Providing calm support.
- Participating in behavioural management procedures.
- Chaperoning clinician.
- Practising patient rapport.
- Monitoring.
- Knowing basic life support.
- Initiating patient rescue.

The dental nurse must:
- monitor the patient during sedation
- have a specific assignment in the event of an emergency
- have current knowledge of the emergency trolley inventory
- be able to demonstrate basic life support skills.

The Family Dentist as a Sedationist

> A dentist must only use conscious sedation for which he or she has been specifically trained and found competent.

It is important that conscious sedation is used as an extension of behavioural management techniques. With that in mind it is assumed that the dental sedationist will use techniques appropriate to the individual child, as described in previous chapters. In addition, there are specific supplementary roles and responsibilities relating to conscious sedation.

Key Roles and Duties

Dental sedationist
- Assessing the dental and medical health of the child.
- Gaining informed consent.
- Prescribing and administering sedation.
- Monitoring sedated child.
- Post-procedurally caring for and discharging child.

The dental sedationist must:
- understand the pharmacokinetics and the pharmacodynamics of the sedative drug being used

- be trained in at least basic life support
- be able to rescue a child whose level of sedation becomes deeper than planned
- have adequate ongoing experience
- demonstrate evidence of continuing education and professional development in paediatric dental sedation.

Preparing the Facilities

The dental environment must be child-friendly and welcoming to both the anxious child and their escort. Sedation in children must only be performed in an environment where facilities, personnel and equipment to manage paediatric emergency situations are immediately available. Children should be sedated as near as possible to the location of the operative dental procedure. It is extremely unwise to allow a child to be sedated at home prior to attending for a procedure since the prescribing dentist has no control over the dose or the means of transport used to convey the child to the practice. The dental surgery should be large enough to allow access for the staff all around the child patient.

What you need
The following items of equipment should be available in all dental surgeries whether or not conscious sedation is offered:
- basic life support equipment
- oxygen
- suction
- resuscitation bags and masks
- airways, in a range of sizes.

Monitoring
Monitoring begins when the sedative drug is administered and continues until the child is fully recovered.

Minimum alert clinical monitoring
The minimal monitoring standard is regular clinical assessment of:
- the level of consciousness
- respiratory rate and pattern
- pulse rate
- skin and mucosal colour.

During conscious sedation the patient should respond to verbal commands. Whenever you ask the patient to perform an action and they do this during the procedure you are checking that their level of consciousness is appropriate. Traditional methods of monitoring sedated paediatric patients include visual observation of skin colour, depth and rate of respiration, measuring pulse and blood pressure and listening to heart and breath sounds using a precordial stethoscope.

- Listen to the respiratory rate and pattern to ensure that there are no obstructions.
- Observe the chest to assess the depth and rate of respiration.
- Monitor the pulse rate by either feeling the radial pulse or, more accurately, the carotid pulse.
- Measuring the pulse can also be a useful means of assessing anxiety: pulse rates increase if patients are becoming anxious.
- Skin tones differ between individuals and so it is the changes in colour during treatment that are more useful to observe, rather than the actual skin colour.

What is Hypoxaemia?

Hypoxaemia is defined as a low partial pressure of oxygen in the blood. It may be caused by:
- failure of oxygen supply
- pulmonary disease
- cardiovascular collapse
- hyperventilation
- apnoea (cessation of breathing)
- airway obstruction.

The quicker the dental team is alerted to a fall in oxygen saturation (hypoxaemia) the better.

The following simple steps can usually prevent prolonged hypoxaemia, especially when the level of sedation meets the contemporary definition.
- Stop.
- Open the airway (to do this, adjust the child's posture by lifting his or her mandible up from his or her chest).
- Clear the airway (to do this, check that no dental materials have been aspirated or are causing an obstruction).
- Ensure verbal communication is maintained.
- If, after all this, the child is clearly conscious, check the pulse oximetry probe – it may be a false alarm!
- If hypoxaemia doesn't immediately improve, START BASIC LIFE SUPPORT PROCEDURES.

It is vital to have trained personnel skilled in conscious sedation so as to monitor the safety and well-being of the sedated child dental patient. However, hypoxaemia can occur before there are detectable changes in vital signs or skin and mucosal colour and symptoms may not become clinically evident until dangerously low levels of oxygen tension develop. For this reason, conscious sedative techniques, with the exception of nitrous oxide inhalation sedation, require pulse oximetry.

Pulse Oximetry

Pulse oximetry directly measures arterial haemoglobin oxygen saturation and, as such, has revolutionised modern monitoring procedures. It is non-invasive, using a sensor probe placed on the patient's finger or ear lobe, which has an red light source to detect the relative difference in the absorption of light between saturated and desaturated haemoglobin during arterial pulsation. Adequate oxygenation of the tissues occurs above 95%, while oxygen saturations lower than this are considered hypoxaemic. In room air a child's normal oxygen saturation (SaO_2) is 97% to 100%.

Pulse oximetry may also be used to engage the child in the dental procedure by assisting the dentist to focus the child's attention (a form of distraction). By asking the child to take deep breaths, and see if they can get "100%", they are given something to do. Some practitioners also tell stories during the procedure and incorporate the monitor's heart beat sounds into the tale.

Capnography

The pulse oximeter probe is sensitive to patient movement, relative hypothermia, ambient light and abnormal haemoglobinaemias, so false readings can occur, particularly when supplemental oxygen is given. Therefore, the role of carbon dioxide monitoring (capnography), as an adjunct to pulse oxymetry and alert clinical observation, is under increasing scrutiny. Capnography monitors respiratory ventilation with greater sensitivity and accuracy than pulse oximetry. Indeed, end-tidal carbon dioxide monitoring is fast becoming the preferred method of detecting apnoea. The technique has gradually developed and now non-invasive nasal cannulae can be used. However, it is a technique that has not as yet found widespread use in paediatric dental sedation.

Do you need electronic monitoring for nitrous oxide inhalation sedation?
No! Alert clinical monitoring is enough when nitrous oxide is used to sedate a child in accordance with the GDC definition

So when do you need electronic monitoring?
For all types of conscious sedation EXCEPT nitrous oxide inhalation sedation.

Key Points

- Alert clinical monitoring is acceptable for nitrous oxide inhalation sedation.
- All other forms of sedation need (at least) pulse oximetry in addition to this.
- Make sure all the equipment is there, including the dental materials, before the sedation is begun.
- STAY CHAPARONED AT ALL TIMES.

Recovery

A quiet area or recovery room is needed in different circumstances. First, for patients who have been sedated, while the sedative agent is taking effect. Secondly, following conscious sedation, whilst the patient is recovering. Few primary care dental facilities have the luxury of a quiet room, although many dentists would desire this for themselves during a busy working day! The idea behind a "quiet room" is to provide an area where the child can be supervised and monitored whilst they are becoming increasingly sedated. Such an area is essential if oral sedation, for example, is provided. With some clever scheduling, this room can be used later to monitor children who are then recovering following the sedative procedure. A suitably qualified member of staff should be present at all times, although a one-way mirrored window, if the monitors and child are in easy sight of the team, might be less anxiety-provoking. If no separate quiet room is available then the child must be sedated and recovered in the dental chair and the appointment scheduling lengthened to facilitate this.

Quiet room specifications
Check list:
- adequate access for the dental team around the child
- ready availability of resuscitation equipment and drugs
- suction
- oxygen
- pulse oximeter with audible alarm (minimum)
- telephone
- soft easy chair for parent to hold child in their lap if appropriate
- chair or bed to allow head-down tilt
- good lighting

- soft lighting
- child-friendly decoration
- separate from the waiting room
- in the immediate vicinity of the whole dental team should an emergency arise.

Drug monitoring

Dental surgeries are often situated in community clinics or near to main thoroughfares. Sedative drugs (and needles that can be used intravenously) appeal to thieves and so these have to be securely stored, even during the working day whilst the surgery is staffed. Sadly, the often-stressful nature of the profession and the many problems that can arise in any small business team, can even lead to drug misuse by staff. Therefore, all drugs must be securely stored in a lockable cabinet and the stock inventory regularly monitored and updated.

Special precautions when using nitrous oxide inhalation sedation

In addition to taking steps to ensure routine safe storage, prescription and handling of drugs and needles in the dental surgery, extra care must be provided when nitrous oxide is used (Fig 9-1).

Sedationists using nitrous oxide inhalation sedation must ensure that
- Only dedicated dental machines are used.
- Equipment must be regularly maintained.
- Installed machines must have non–interchangeable colour-coded pipelines fitted with a low pressure warning system with an audible alarm.
- The use and storage of any anaesthetic gas, such as nitrous oxide, must comply with The Control of Substances Hazardous to Health (COSHH) Regulations 1999.
- Adequate scavenging is provided (see below).

Safety features found in portable dental inhalation sedation units

A number of safety features are incorporated within portable dental inhalation sedation machines used to administer nitrous oxide inhalation sedation. These include:

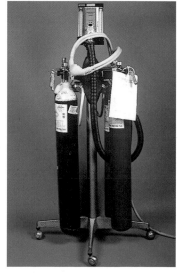

Fig 9-1 Dedicated nitrous oxide inhalation sedation.

- pin valves to prevent accidental reversal of oxygen and nitrous oxide tanks
- oxygen tanks colour-coded black
- nitrous oxide tanks colour-coded blue
- nitrous oxide cut-out if oxygen flow stops
- regulated delivery of no less than 30% oxygen.

Different pin systems for each gaseous agent combined with the tank colour-coding system ensure that oxygen and nitrous oxide cylinders cannot be confused and the wrong tanks mistakenly fitted to the machine. By guaranteeing that a minimum percentage (30%) of oxygen must be delivered and that the machine will stop delivering nitrous oxide if the oxygen cylinder is not functioning, it is almost impossible to oversedate a patient.

The equipment should be set up and checked prior to the patient's arrival. This includes a full test of the machine including the gas supply, nosepiece, tubing and scavenging. Ideally, the correct size nosepiece should be chosen at the assessment visit. The patient's medical history and understanding of the procedure should be rechecked. The nosepiece is positioned by the patient and tightened to prevent leaks.

In addition, all circuitry and equipment should be either disposable or autoclavable to ensure continued high standards of cross-infection control.

Scavenging is essential with nitrous oxide

Scavenging is the collection and removal of vented anaesthetic gases. The amount of anaesthetic gas supplied usually far exceeds the amount necessary for the patient, so control of occupational exposure to nitrous oxide in the dental surgery is a serious concern. However, with effective scavenging of waste gases there are no adverse effects. The recommended limit is an average of 100 parts per million over an eight hour exposure period. Adequate ventilation and scavenging equipment is therefore strongly recommended and a number of other methods are suggested to ensure that nitrous oxide levels remain as low as possible (Fig 9-2).

Possible Toxicity of Nitrous Oxide to the Dental Team

Risks include:
- liver disease
- miscarriage
- bone marrow suppression
- addiction

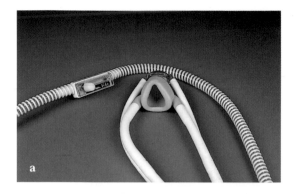

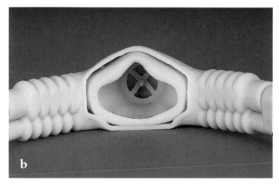

Fig 9-2 a, b Examples of a nitrous oxide inhalation sedation scavenging nosepiece.

- carcinoma
- birth defects
- depression of vitamin B12 activity.

To Control Occupational Exposure

- Use a properly maintained gas delivery system.
- Use a scavenging nosepiece (no air-entrainment valve should be used).
- Use a positive pressure gas evacuation system.
- Minimise speech by the patient.
- Use a rubber dam.
- Use fans to waft the nitrous oxide gas away from the dentist and dental nurse.

Practical Tips

- A dentist must only use conscious sedation for which they have been specifically trained and found competent.
- Every member of the dental team has a role in the success and safety of paediatric dental sedation.
- Train the team.
- Work as a team.
- Contact a respected organisation that offers conscious sedation training before offering it to patients.
- Remember to ensure the health and safety of your staff as well as your patient.
- Always have a chaperone.
- Look after the health and safety of the dental team. Comply with COSHH regulations in respect of nitrous oxide pollution and gas safety.
- Alert clinical monitoring is acceptable for nitrous oxide inhalation sedation.
- All other forms of sedation need (at least) pulse oximetry in addition to this alert clinical monitoring.

Further Reading

Anderson JA, Vann WFJ. Respiratory monitoring during pediatric sedation: pulse oximetry and capnography. Ped Dent 1988;10:94–101.

Health and Safety Advisory Committee, Health and Safety Executive, Anaesthetic Agents: Controlling Exposure Under COSSH. London: HMSO, 1995.

Scottish Intercollegiate Guideline Network (SIGN). Safe Sedation of Children Undergoing Diagnostic and Therapeutic Procedures. National Clinical Guideline Number 58. www.sign.ac.uk.

Standards in Conscious Sedation for Dentistry. Report of an Independent Expert Working Group. October 2000. Available from The Society for the Advancement of Anaesthesia in Dentistry (SAAD), 53 Wimpole Street, London W1G 8YH. www.saaduk.org

Whitcher CE, Zimmerman DC, Tonn EM, Piziali RL. Control of occupational exposure to nitrous oxide in the dental operatory. J Amer Dent Assoc 1977;95:763–776.

Chapter 10

Conscious Sedation 4: What to Use and How to Use It

Aim

The main aim of this chapter is to review sedative drugs and techniques that can be used by general dental practitioners. Particular emphasis will be placed on nitrous oxide inhalation sedation since this is the most common technique used for paediatric dental sedation. A secondary aim is to give dentists an overview of the benzodiazepine, midazolam, since this is becoming increasingly used in specialist referral centres.

Outcome

The dental sedationist and their team should:
- become familiar with inhalational, oral and intravenous routes of administration and be aware of the relative pros and cons of each
- know the indications and contraindications for nitrous oxide inhalation sedation
- understand how to develop their own nitrous oxide inhalation sedation technique
- gain an insight into the use of midazolam.

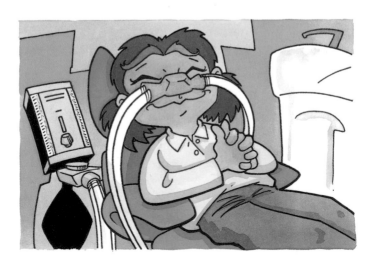

Fig 10-1
Sedated child.

Introduction

Conscious sedation helps to reduce fear and anxiety and enables the anxious but potentially cooperative child not only to accept dental treatment but also to cope better with dental care in future (Fig 10-1). Although broad aspects of dental sedation will be touched upon, this text is intended to assist colleagues working in primary dental care within the United Kingdom and will therefore concentrate on those sedative agents and techniques that are the most likely to be safely and successfully used for child patients within that sector.

Routes of Administering Sedative Drugs to Children

The following routes are used most commonly to administer drugs that produce sedation in dental practice:
- inhalational
- oral
- rectal
- intramuscular
- intravenous.

Inhalational
Nitrous oxide gas has been used extensively in dental practice and is well noted for its analgesic and anaesthetic properties.

Nitrous oxide
- Is a very weak analgesic and so requires concomitant local anaesthetic agents.
- Involves the use of low concentrations of nitrous oxide gas in combination with oxygen for inhalational sedation in conscious patients.
- The technique incorporates behavioural management and hypnotic suggestion.
- Was described as early as 1889 when it was used during cavity preparation in Liverpool Dental School.
- Has been described in detail in the dental literature.

Oral
A survey of current premedication trends in paediatric dental practice in the USA found the oral route to be the most popular in paediatric dentistry. Advantages of this route are:
- ease of administration
- decreased incidence of allergic reaction.

However, major disadvantages include:
* prolonged onset and duration of action
* unpredictable gastric absorption
* dependence on the compliance of the patient
* difficulty in determining appropriate dosages.

Rectal
Although the rectal route has been reported to be successful in paediatric dentistry literature, especially in Scandanavia, it has not found widespread acceptance in the United Kingdom. This is probably because an enema is required, a procedure best performed in hospital rather than a dental practice.

Intramuscular
The intramuscular technique has several advantages over the oral route in that it allows:
* a more rapid onset of effect
* more reliable absorption of the agent into the circulation.

However:
* it is difficult to titrate medications with sufficient accuracy to obtain a predictable response
* an intramuscular injection is needed! This can be distressing for an already anxious child
* many dental practitioners are not familiar with intramuscular injection techniques.

Intravenous
The intravenous route of drug administration is the most effective method of ensuring predictable and adequate sedation of rapid onset and short duration in adults.

However:
* this requires venepuncture!
* children have such small veins and chubby hands
* it is generally reserved for anxious adolescents who are mature enough to accept it and adult dental patients
* this is the least well researched route in paediatric dental sedation and so is not generally recommended for use in primary dental care settings.

Drugs Used to Sedate Children for Dentistry

The commonest drugs used when anxious children are undergoing dental treatment under conscious sedation are local anaesthesia and nitrous oxide.

Nitrous oxide inhalation sedation
Properties of nitrous oxide
Nitrous oxide has only a mild sedative effect so inhalation sedation is more reliant on operator suggestion than other sedative techniques. The operator's ability to relax and talk the patient through the process is as critical as the drug itself. In this sense inhalation sedation augments other behavioural management techniques it does not replace them (Fig 10-2).

Nitrous oxide gas:
• has a sweet odour that is pleasant to inhale
• is non-irritant to both the lungs and nasal passages.

Poor tissue solubility ensures the effects are of rapid onset and that recovery is fast. Remember, children can become hypoxic much more readily than adults and so if too little oxygen is delivered they can be rendered unconscious.

How well does nitrous oxide inhalation sedation work?
In the last fifteen years there have been many studies to determine the efficacy of nitrous oxide/oxygen sedation. Double blind cross over trials undertaken by different authors in children have shown that nitrous oxide:
• is a very effective conscious sedation technique when used in combination with behavioural therapy
• reduces mild to moderate anxious and uncooperative behaviour
• facilitates coping across sequential visits
• reduces the gag reflex
• BUT is less effective in the management of patients with severe anxiety and uncooperative behaviour (Fig 10-3).

Indications and contraindications of nitrous oxide inhalation sedation in dental practice
Inhalation sedation requires the patient to be moderately cooperative and to understand what is being done. Patients who are too young to understand or who have severe intellectual impairments should not be treated. While there is no absolute age bar most studies have found patients less than 4 years of age unable to cope.
Severe anxiety may also affect a child's ability to cooperate; if you are unable

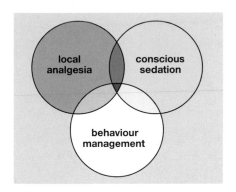

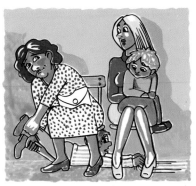

Fig 10-2 The association between local anaesthesia, conscious sedation and behavioural management.

Fig 10-3 Nitrous oxide inhalation sedation is most effective in moderately anxious children.

to carry out an intraoral examination at the assessment visit it is unlikely that cooperation will be adequate for treatment with inhalation sedation.

The complexity of the procedure to be undertaken must also be considered. Traumatic or long or complicated procedures may be better treated under general anaesthetic for some children - for example, the removal of four first permanent molars.

Because inhalation sedation depends upon a patent nasal airway, any nasal blockage is a contraindication. For temporary obstructions (a cold or hay fever, for example) treatment can be rescheduled but if the obstruction is permanent an alternative form of sedation is required.

There are a number of other conditions where inhalation sedation is inappropriate and these are indicated in Table 10-1.

Adverse reactions to nitrous oxide
Nitrous oxide inhalation sedation is the best researched and carries less risk of complication than other sedative agents used in paediatric dentistry. Nevertheless, just like any drug, nitrous oxide is not without adverse reactions.

Some of the (rare) reported adverse affect are listed below:
• hypoxia
• malignant hyperpyrexia (controversial)
• loss of protective reflexes

- nausea and vomiting
- bone marrow depression (B12)
- diffusion hypoxia
- pressure/volume effects (ear)
- psychological effects:
  - euphoria,
  - hallucinations,
  - claustrophobia
- fire.

(from: J Am Dent Assoc 1984;108:213-219)

Toxicity of nitrous oxide to dentists and their assistants
Prolonged exposure or multiple short exposures to nitrous oxide can result in depression of vitamin B12 activity. Dental surgeons are particularly at risk since they are exposed to high concentrations in the confined space of the dental surgery, especially if scavenging is inadequate. It has a number of other side effects, including an increased risk of miscarriage. The most significant finding in these studies was the importance of scavenging, since all effects

Table 10-1 **Indications and contraindications for inhalation sedation**

Indication	Contraindication
• Mild to moderate dental anxiety	• Extreme anxiety
• Marked gag reflex	• Unable to understand (too young or intellectual impairment)
• Traumatic procedure in cooperative patient	• Nasal blockage
• Needle phobia	• Severe psychiatric disorders
• Orthodontic extractions in anxious patients	• First trimester of pregnancy
• Multiple quadrant dentistry in young patients	• Chronic bronchitis
	• Claustrophobia
	• Myasthema gravis
	• Multiple sclerosis

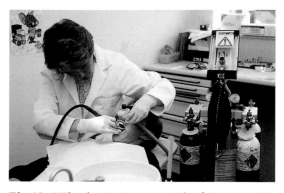

Fig 10-4 The dentist is most at risk of nitrous oxide toxicity.

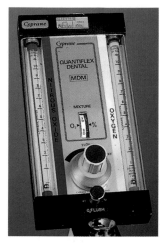

Fig 10-5 Portable dedicated dental inhalation sedation machine.

were more apparent in groups who had worked with no scavenging. Scavenging (Fig 10-4) is discussed in Chapter 9.

Technique for nitrous oxide inhalation sedation
In paediatric dentistry nitrous oxide concentrations of up to 30% (i.e. 70% oxygen) are the most commonly used to produce the desired sedation but the final concentration has to be titrated to obtain the optimal effect in each individual child (Fig 10-5).

The mixture is set to 100% oxygen and the flow rate adjusted to match the patient's tidal volume. Nitrous oxide is then titrated to match the patient's needs, starting with 10% nitrous oxide for one minute. If necessary this is increased to 20% nitrous oxide for one minute. If sedation is not sufficient 5% increases may be used. It is possible to give 50% nitrous oxide but it is unusual for patients to require more than 35%.

Throughout the procedure suggestion and reassurance is given. This is as important as the nitrous oxide, which makes the patient more susceptible to the operator's instructions. The exact nature of the suggestion varies between operators – for example, some describe the pleasant sensations that the nitrous oxide may produce; others will tell the patient stories or ask them to choose a favourite place and imagine they are there.

Table 10-2 **How to carry out nitrous oxide inhalation sedation**

Titrate the concentration of nitrous oxide	• Dry room air contains 21% Oxygen • Some children might exhibit signs of unconsciousness or light general anaesthesia at 40% concentrations of nitrous oxide • Titrate in 5% concentrations at 3–5 minute intervals • Seldom need go beyond 30% nitrous oxide

Inhalation sedation (IHS) method: monitor response	• KEEP TALKING
	• Ensure the child avoids mouth breathing
	• Continue behavioural management e.g.
	  – Tell-Show-Do (TSD)
	  –Positive reinforcement
	  –Acclimatisation
	• MAXIMUM when child reports "tingling" or starts giggling/ becomes overexcited.
	• STOP if ears ringing or sore head

When the appropriate level of sedation is reached treatment can start. Ensure that the patient continues to breathe through the nose, not the mouth during treatment, to maintain adequate sedation and limit the amount of nitrous oxide that is released. Turning the dial to 100% oxygen and having the patient breathe this for a minimum of two minutes starts the recovery process. This ensures that nitrous oxide is scavenged and not released into the atmosphere. The patient should be allowed to breathe without the nosepiece for five minutes and is released from the surgery for a further fifteen minutes. The technique is summarised in Table 10-2.

Benzodiazepines
The benzodiazepines have been extensively used by both the medical and dental professions. They are:
• anxiolytic
• hypnotic
• anticonvulsant
• muscle relaxants.

IMPORTANTLY
- Benzodiazepines produce an antegrade amnesia.
- Although the specific mechanism underlying such diverse actions remains unclear it is believed that the benzodiazepines exert an anxiolytic effect by increasing the glycine inhibitory neurotransmitter. Their ability to act as a hypnotic is related to occupation of the benzodiazepine receptors found exclusively in the central nervous system and consequent gamma-aminobutyric acid (GABA) accumulation.

Midazolam

Midazolam has superseded diazepam for use in dentistry. Whilst the use of intravenous midazolam has been widely reported in adults, there are few studies to support its routine use in the dental management of anxious children.

Oral midazolam

Studies have produced conflicting results and are further confounded by the use of restraints and co-sedatives. Oral midazolam reaches the systemic circulation via the portal circulation; this decreases the drug's bioavailability, necessitating a higher oral dosage compared to intravenous administration. Midazolam is now available in hospitals in a blackcurrant-flavoured solution, although not widespread within the United Kingdom. It is therefore used as the intravenous formulation mixed with fruit juice to hide its terrible taste.

Intranasal midazolam

Intranasal administration of midazolam produces a sedative effect within five minutes of administration. Studies using intranasal midazolam in paediatric dental patients are few in number and have involved few subjects but have shown that amnesia can be induced. The administered dose is limited by the volume of the solution, since large volumes can cause coughing, sneezing and expulsion of part of the drug. There have been reports of occasional respiratory depression and transient burning discomfort affecting the nasal mucosa.

The benzodiazepine reversal agent: flumazenil

The introduction of the specific benzodiazepine reversal agent, flumazenil (Anexate®, Roche), has further promoted midazolam as a safe and reliable agent for induction of anaesthesia, conscious sedation and intravenous infusion. Some authors have compared it to the already established opioid antagonist naloxone The duration of action is 15 to 140 minutes and is dose dependent. Intravenous doses are given incrementally until an effect is produced but oral administration has also been reported. However, the half-life of flumazenil seems to be shorter than the benzodiazepine and so resedation has been reported. Postoperative anxiety has also been reported although carefully titrated doses might avoid this undesirable stress response.

Paediatric product licence
Neither flumazenil nor midazolam has a product licence to sanction their administration to children. Furthermore, studies where midazolam has been used in the paediatric population have used the drug either in combination with other agents or using a mixture of routes. The unpredictable onset of effect and prolonged recovery of other benzodiazepines make them unattractive to paediatric dental sedation.

Other drugs used in paediatric specialist practice
Other drug groups used for paediatric dental sedation include sedative hypnotics, psychosedatives and narcotics. Paediatric dentistry specialists, mainly in North America, have generally reported their use. These agents include chloral hydrate, hydroxyzine hydrochloride, pethidine and anaesthetic agents such as propofol and ketamine. This book is designed to facilitate child management in primary dental care in the United Kingdom and so these drugs will not be explored further in this text.

Polypharmacy: not a good idea
The use of drug combinations or premixed drug cocktails is generally best avoided because of the increased risk of side effects. Respiratory depression is more likely to occur when more that one sedative agent is administered.

Practical Tips

- United Kingdom sedationists MUST always comply with the contemporary definition of conscious sedation.
- In nitrous oxide inhalation sedation, the operator's ability to relax and talk the patient through the process is as crucial as the drug itself.
- Remember that local anaesthesia is also a drug!

Further Reading

Duncan GH, Moore P. Nitrous oxide and the dental patient: a review of adverse reactions. J Am Dent Assoc 1984;108:213-219.

Ferguson S, Ball AJ. Sedation and sedative drugs in paediatrics. [Review] [18 refs]. Br J Hosp Med 1996;55:611–615.

Roberts GJ, Gibson A, Porter J, de Zoysa S. Relative analgesia: an evaluation of the efficacy and safety. Br Dent J 1979;146:177–182.

United Kingdom National Clinical Guidelines in Paediatric Dentistry. Managing anxious children: the use of conscious sedation in paediatric dentistry. Int J Paed Dent 2002;12:325–372.

Veerkamp JS, Gruythuysen RJ, Hoogstraten J, van Amerongen WE. Anxiety reduction with nitrous oxide: a permanent solution? ASDC J Dent Child 1995;62:44–48.

Chapter 11
General Anaesthesia

Aim

In this chapter we will review the use of general anaesthesia in respect of current legislation in the United Kingdom and explore its role in contemporary paediatric dental management.

Outcome

At the end of this chapter practitioners should be able to:
- assess a child's dental needs
- understand the reasons for considering the use of general anaesthesia
- refer correctly to the most appropriate specialist centre
- understand the importance of follow-up preventive care to reduce the need for a future repeat general anaesthesia.

Introduction

Patients who are too apprehensive to undergo dental treatment solely with local analgesia may be managed with a skilful combination of local anaesthesia and sedation. Indeed, nitrous oxide inhalation sedation offers a strong alternative to general anaesthesia but it is not always potent enough to treat the recalcitrant child. Sometimes a general anaesthetic is necessary with a "pre-coopera-tive" child or because of the presence of acute infection, dental disease in several quadrants or a medical or learning disability (Fig 11-1).

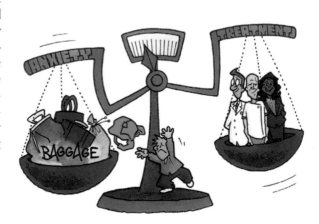

Fig 11-1

"Pre-cooperative" children

We learned from previous chapters that the cooperation of a child is dependent on their level of emotional maturity, previous experience and on family influence, particularly maternal attitude towards dental treatment. Toddlers are generally "pre-cooperative" - they have very limited communication skills and few ways of expressing their anxieties and fears. Their ability to accept dental treatment is limited. When they feel unsure or threatened they try to escape and usually do this by crying. This crying is an aversive stimulus that prompts the listener to act - for example, the parent intervenes and stops whatever is making the child cry (Fig 11-2).

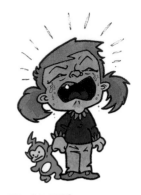

Fig 11-2 The precooperative child with toothache may need a general anaesthetic.

Why is general anaesthesia so commonly used in the United Kingdom?

An upturn in general anaesthesia activity was reported in north-west England in 1998, attributable to more children five years of age and younger having untreated caries due to the combined effect of an increase in caries and fewer decayed teeth being filled. Indeed, there is a clear correlation between the level of social deprivation and the numbers of decayed, missing and filled teeth in children. Children, especially those of pre-school age, who have the highest risk of dental caries are often not registered with a dentist, and consequently may not be receiving the intensive preventive and operative care that they need. Mothers of socially deprived children tend to delay taking their child to a dentist until their child is experiencing pain and are more likely to demand extractions. Therefore, dentists are still commonly presented with a child in pain who is attending their practice for the first time, and for whom extraction under a general anaesthetic appears to be the only option.

What is General Anaesthesia?

General anaesthesia is defined as "a controlled state of unconsciousness accompanied by a loss of protective reflexes, including the ability to maintain an airway independently and respond purposefully to physical stimulation or verbal command". Thus general anaesthesia is any technique that produces a degree of depression of the central nervous system greater than

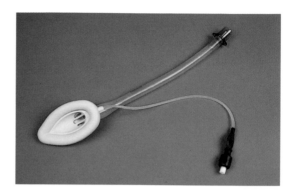

Fig 11-3 A laryngeal mask.

that covered by the definition of conscious sedation. The respiratory function of a patient who is under a general anaesthetic is compromised since they are unconscious and unable to maintain the patency of their own airway. To overcome this an anaesthetist positions the patient in such a manner that the airway is maintained or uses Geudel airways, nasopharyngeal tubes or endotracheal intubation. In modern practice, laryngeal masks are increasingly popular [Fig 11-3]. General anaesthesia can be induced and maintained using inhalational or intravenous agents and there is a plethora of such techniques available, tailored to the suit each operative procedure and the needs of the individual patient.

Contemporary United Kingdom Legislation

The Royal Collage of Anaesthetists has advised that general anaesthesia should be strictly limited to those patients and clinical situations in which local anaesthesia with or without sedation is not an option. Moreover, the General Dental Council has announced amendments to its regulations precluding all but anaesthetists who conform to set parameters laid down by the General Medical Council from administering general anaesthesia for dental treatment. The referring dental practitioner for each case is obliged:
- to give a clear written justification for the use of general anaesthesia
- to take a full medical history
- to explain to patients and parents the risks associated with general anaesthesia
- to outline alternative methods of treatment
- to provide a comprehensive referral letter
- to keep a copy of their letter of referral.

In summary
- Concern has grown about dental general anaesthesia for many years.
- There has been increasing restrictions on its delivery.
- This has led to a reduction of its use in general dental practice and reduced numbers overall.
- Many GDPs have stopped providing a general anaesthesia service.
- Patients are referred elsewhere for treatment under general anaesthesia.

The cumulative effect of these recommendations is to remove general anaesthesia from nearly all general dental practice settings. Consequently, more children with caries are being referred to the community dental service and to hospital-based paediatric dental units.

Reasons for Child Dental Extractions under General Anaesthesia

A study of referrals to Leicestershire Community Dental Service General Anaesthesia Facility found 25% of the children were not only attending the referring GDP for the first time ever, but were also presenting with acute pain. General anaesthesia simplifies the extraction procedure in young children as it minimises the need for cooperation.

Reasons for extracting children's teeth under general anaesthesia include:
- dental pain
- facial swelling
- extractions in multiple quadrants
- patient anxiety
- the young age of the patient ("pre-cooperative")
- poor record of attendance
- history of poor cooperation in the past
- parental choice.

Extract or restore?
In the United Kingdom, even though dental treatment for children is provided free of charge under the National Health Service, the general public have given child dental health low priority. The primary dentition in particular is considered to have little value, resulting in a demand for extraction rather than restorative therapy. Because of this, dental practitioners in the United Kingdom have been heavily reliant on extractions under general anaesthesia, resulting in space loss, despite the proven efficacy of primary prevention and early caries diagnosis (Fig 11-4).

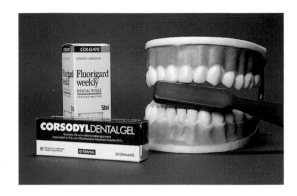

Fig 11-4 Prevention is better than cure.

In Scotland, for example, a culture of dental extractions under general anaesthesia has become established over many years, and accepted by both families and dentists as the principal method of dental treatment of carious primary teeth. This high level of extractions cannot be entirely attributed to the high level of caries in this population. Indeed, if the caries experience of 5- and 6-year-old Scottish children is compared with similar areas in Europe, decayed and filled rates are very similar but more teeth are extracted.

Problems with the early extraction of primary teeth include:
- delayed eruption of the permanent successors
- premolar crowding
- difficulty chewing
- aesthetics.

Restoration of primary molars can also be undertaken under general anaesthesia by referral to a specialist paediatric dentistry unit. This is a longer procedure, requiring intubation, commonly with a laryngeal mask. This type of oral rehabilitation is therefore usually carried out in a day surgery unit based in a children's hospital. The availability of this type of service, though more common in other parts of the world, is limited both by cost and by the number of hospital-based paediatric dentistry specialists in the United Kingdom.

Irrespective of the type of treatment offered under general anaesthesia, without a preventive programme many children will later undergo a further general anaesthesia for dental extractions.

The Problem of Repeat General Anaesthesia

The problem of attendance for repeat referral is a serious one; between 23% and 31% of children subsequently require a further general anaesthesia for dental treatment. Indeed, MacCormack and Kinirons (1998) report that children below four years of age have the highest risk. The failure to extract minimally carious teeth at the child's first general anaesthesia visit might be founded in a misplaced optimism and a wish to save these teeth but, in a recent study, such an approach might have accounted for 85% of repeat general anaesthesias. Instead, the authors suggest that more children could be offered restorations under general anaesthesia in a day surgery unit. There is also evidence to suggest that even when all carious teeth are extracted or restored the first permanent molars subsequently develop caries when they erupt and as such may still necessitate a further general anaesthetic if anxiety is not ameliorated.

The Importance of a Thorough Dental Assessment

The scope of the general anaesthesia service does not always include a radiographic examination or a formal dental assessment by a paediatric dentist. Indeed, the dentist at the general anaesthesia centre usually has no prior knowledge of the child's ability to cooperate with dental treatment. Whilst parents might be able to assist in predicting the behaviour of their child, the assessment of anxiety in children is even more challenging at this late stage. A specialist paediatric dentist is perhaps better able to perform such an assessment and better skilled in the selection of those children who should be offered conscious sedation. Indeed, referral to a specialist screening service has been shown to lead to an increased number of extractions, resulting in a reduction in the need for a repeat general anaesthesia. Such an assessment is also more likely to favour the use of alternatives to general anaesthesia such as local anaesthesia and sedation.

Assessment prior to general anaesthesia

In many Community Dental Services and Hospital Dental Services, pregeneral anaesthesia assessment clinics have been initiated with patients attending prior to any subsequent appointment for general anaesthesia extractions. In other areas, the operating dentist runs a formal pre-assessment clinic for all general anaesthesia patients. In some parts of England, pregeneral anaesthesia assessment clinics conducted by the Community Dental Service have been used to reduce the number of patients receiving a general anaesthetic. In addition, they have sought to ensure that the anaesthetist has a satisfactory medical history and that the dental officer undertaking the extractions has satisfactory clinical information to undertake the proposed care.

Risk Associated With General Anaesthesia

Cases of mortality following dental general anaesthesia for children have been instrumental in United Kingdom reviews of provision of this service. Although deaths are relatively rare, morbidity is commonplace. A recent study in Lancashire investigated the effects on children of tooth extraction under general anaesthesia. For the 80 children of 2 to 15 years of age, 92% complained of symptoms associated with the procedure. Twenty percent of children were clearly distressed during the induction, and 33% during recovery, with continued crying for 39% on the journey home and for 37% once home had been reached. Other symptoms include nausea, sickness and prolonged bleeding. Indeed, some adult dental phobics have identified the effects of a general anaesthesia for dental extractions in childhood as the source of their avoidance of dental care.

Informed Consent for General Anaesthesia

Dentists are obliged to:
- explain the reason for treatment under general anaesthesia
- discuss the alternative treatment options
- gain informed consent.

However, an audit of children referred for general anaesthesia extractions in Scotland showed that a surprising number of parents reported that neither the risks nor the alternatives were discussed. Clearly, many of the referring dentists must have felt that they had fulfilled their obligations in this regard but somehow their message was either inadequate or unmemorable. Therefore, it is essential that dentists clearly document that the risks have been explained and the alternatives discussed. Careful practitioners might wish the parent or guardian to sign the referral documentation to confirm that this information has been both delivered and understood.

What Type of General Anaesthesia? Referral Options

To determine whether the individual can be treated as an outpatient or inpatient depends on:
- the technique used by the anaesthetist

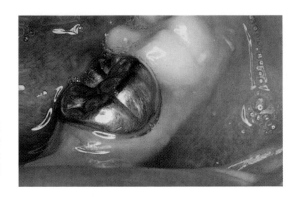

Fig 11-5 Stainless steel crowns last longer than other primary molar restorations when there is interproximal involvement.

- the operative procedure (extraction only or full oral rehabilitation)
- the medical fitness of the patient (for example, a patient who is diabetic or who requires endotracheal intubation generally requires in-patient medical supervision).

When you need a specialist paediatric dentistry service

Paediatric dentistry specialists are common in North America and in some other parts of the world, but the only European Union countries to recognise this speciality are the United Kingdom and Sweden. So what do paediatric dentistry specialists do? In the United Kingdom, these rare beings are mainly, but not exclusively, in the community and hospital services and in academic institutions. One of their key roles is in managing anxious children. Another is providing oral care for children with medically compromising conditions such as leukaemia, organ transplantation, oncology and cardiac defects.

Referral to a specialist paediatric dentistry service should be considered when:
- a medically compromised child is likely to need a general anaesthetic
- oral rehabilitation under general anaesthesia may be more appropriate than extractions only
- the child requiring a general anaesthesia has a dental anomaly (e.g. hypodontia) (Fig 11-5).

Follow-up post general anaesthesia

Since children often feel traumatised by their experience of a general anaesthesia for dental treatment, additional support should be offered to them following the visit. This must include primary prevention to reduce caries risk and thereby prevent a repeat general anaesthetic. However, for some children the general dental practitioner may need to establish links with community-based health support teams to deliver this care since some children may not attend for follow-up appointments in the dental surgery. Indeed, referring dentists may not even need to see these patients themselves, professionals complimentary to dentistry such as a dental therapist, could help to ensure that these children receive the preventive care and support that they require.

Practical Tips

- Perform a thorough dental examination, ideally with radiographs, to ensure that all caries is diagnosed.
- A thorough medical history is essential.
- Discuss the risks and alternatives of general anaesthesia with the parents.
- Ensure informed consent is obtained.
- General anaesthesia referral forms should include not only the parent or guardian consent but also written confirmation from them that the risks have been explained and the options discussed.
- Medically compromised children should be referred to a specialist paediatric dentistry team.
- Ensure the child has a follow-up visit arranged.

Further Reading

General Dental Council. Maintaining Standards: Guidance to Dentists on Professional and Personal Conduct. London, 1997 (revised 1998).

Pine C, McPherson L, McGoldrick P, Hosey MT, Taylor M, MacMillan C, Clinical Resource and Audit Group of the Scottish Executive Health Department. Audit of Reasons for Referral of Children for Dental Extractions under General Anaesthesia (99/42). Dundee and Glasgow, Dental Schools: 2001.

Standards and Guidelines for General Anaesthesia for Dentistry. London, Royal College of Anaesthetists: 1999 (www.rcoa.ac.uk).

References

Bridgman CM, Ashby D, Holloway PJ. An investigation of the effects on children of tooth extraction under general anaesthesia in general dental practice. Br Dent J 1999;186:245-247.

Harrison M, Nutting L. Repeat general anaesthesia for paediatric dentistry. Br Dent J 2000; 189:37-39.

Hosey MT, Robertson I, Bedi R. A review of correspondence to a general dental practice helpline. Prim Dent Care 1995;2:43-46.

MacCormac C, Kinirons M. Reasons for referral of children to a general anaesthetic service in Northern Ireland. Int J Paed Dent 1998;8191-8196.

Royal College of Anaesthetists. Standing Dental Advisory Committee. Report of an Expert Working Party (Chairman: Professor D Poswillo). General Anaesthesia, Sedation and Resuscitation in Dentistry. London, 1990.

The Pre-appointment Letter

Dear XXXX

Please find your dental appointment enclosed.

At this first visit you will be introduced to your dentist, Dr Gummer, who will count your teeth for you. You may even have your teeth made to shine using our engine tooth polishers, Mrs Mop and Mr Buzzy!

We are looking forward to meeting you.

Appendix 2

Patient Information Sheet for Inhalation Sedation

INHALATION SEDATION FOR CHILDREN

Another Group of Associates
High Street
Yourtown

Telephone 0870 000 000
www.anothergroupofassociates.co.uk

Our aim

Our aim is to make children's dentistry as comfortable and as easy as possible. Many children that are referred to us are anxious about receiving dental treatment.

What is Inhalation Sedation?

Inhalation sedation has been used in dentistry for almost forty years. The therapy involves breathing a mixture of oxygen and nitrous oxide (laughing gas) through a cup that fits over the nose. The mixture of gases is then carefully adjusted until the child is relaxed, <u>but not asleep</u>. The aim of inhalation sedation is to produce sedation and relaxation, but not sleep. The child is awake and aware of all the people, surroundings and subsequent dental treatment at all times.

Can Any Child Have Inhalation Sedation?

Inhalation sedation is a very safe technique for most children. We will thoroughly check that your child is suitable to have inhalation sedation.

If There Are Any Changes in Their Medication or Health Status, Let Us Know.

Your child will have to be able to breathe through (his) her nose and so if (he) she has a cold we may have to postpone this particular type of treatment until (he) she has recovered.

Is Inhalation Sedation Safe?

For the patient, Yes.

Scavenging equipment is used to reduce nitrous oxide pollution in the surgery, mostly for the benefit of the dentist and assistants.

Will the Tooth Still Need to be Numbed? Will a Local Anaesthetic (Jab) Still be Necessary?

Yes. Our aim is always to ensure that treatment is comfortable and acceptable. Inhalation sedation is used as part of a process involving the gradual introduction to various dental procedures. Therefore, through the course of treatment your child will become less anxious and should become ready to accept a local anaesthetic.

Are There any Special Instructions Before Treatment?

- Eat and drink normally but avoid a particularly heavy meal (a light meal such as tea and toast is acceptable).
- A parent or guardian must always accompany the child. The parent or guardian does not need to stay with the child during the whole treatment session. Often the child prefers his or her parent or guardian to wait in the waiting room.
- The parent or guardian will be asked to sign a consent form.
- Try to avoid bringing other children with you as they can be a distraction to the anxious child.

How You Can Help in the Treatment of Your Child?

The service that we offer is time consuming not only for us, but also for parents and children. Therefore, we would like to draw your attention to the importance of the prevention of further dental disease and future anxiety.

Here are some of the steps that you can take at home to alleviate your child's anxiety and to reduce the need for lengthy dental procedures.

- Prevent tooth decay by cutting down on the number of sugary snacks and drinks taken between meals.
- Prevent gum disease and tooth decay by brushing teeth efficiently with a small amount of fluoride toothpaste at least twice a day.
- Try to avoid "building-up" the child before the visit with such things as stories and jokes about the dentist from other adults and children.
- Try to show the child YOU are not nervous (even if you are!).

Further Information

Further information can be obtained from The Society for the Advancement of Anaesthesia in Dentistry (SAAD) (www.saaduk.org).

Index

Quintessentials for General Dental Practitioners Series

in 36 volumes

Editor-in-Chief: Professor Nairn H F Wilson

The Quintessentials for General Dental Practitioners Series covers basic princi-
ples and key issues in all aspects of modern dental medicine. Each book can be
read as a stand-alone volume or in conjunction with other books in the series.

Publication date,
approximately

Oral Surgery and Oral Medicine, Editor: John G Meechan

Practical Dental Local Anaesthesia	available
Practical Oral Medicine	Spring 2004
Practical Conscious Sedation	Autumn 2003
Practical Surgical Dentistry	Spring 2004

Imaging, Editor: Keith Horner

Interpreting Dental Radiographs	available
Panoramic Radiology	Autumn 2003
Twenty-first Century Dental Imaging	Autumn 2004

Periodontology, Editor: Iain L C Chapple

Understanding Periodontal Diseases: Assessment and Diagnostic Procedures in Practice	available
Decision-Making for the Periodontal Team	Autumn 2003
Successful Periodontal Therapy – A Non-Surgical Approach	Autumn 2003
Periodontal Management of Children, Adolescents and Young Adults	Autumn 2003
Periodontal Medicine in Practice	Spring 2004

Implantology, Editor: Lloyd J Searson

Implants for the General Practitioner	Spring 2004
Managing Orofacial Pain in General Dental Practice	Spring 2004

Endodontics, Editor: John M Whitworth

Rational Root Canal Treatment in Practice	available
Managing Endodontic Failure in Practice	Autumn 2003
Managing Dental Trauma in Practice	Autumn 2003
Managing the Vital Pulp in Practice	Autumn 2004

Prosthodontics, Editor: P Finbarr Allen

Teeth for Life for Older Adults	available
Complete Dentures – from Planning to Problem Solving	Autumn 2003
Removable Partial Dentures – A Systematic Approach	Autumn 2003
Fixed Prosthodontics for the General Dental Practitioner	Autumn 2003
Occlusion: A Theoretical and Team Approach	Autumn 2004

Operative Dentistry, Editor: Paul A Brunton

Decision-Making in Operative Dentistry	available
Applied Dental Materials in Operative Dentistry	Spring 2003
Aesthetic Dentistry	Autumn 2003
Successful Indirect Restorations in General Practice	Spring 2004

Paediatric Dentistry/Orthodontics, Editor: Marie Therese Hosey

Child Taming: How to Cope with Children in Dental Practice	Spring 2003
Paediatric Cariology	Autumn 2003
Treatment Planning for the Developing Dentition	Autumn 2003

General Dentistry and Practice Management, Editor: Raj Rattan

The Business of Dentistry	available
Risk Management in General Dental Practice	Autumn 2003
Practice Management for the Dental Team	Autumn 2003
Application of Information Technology in General Dental Practice	Spring 2004
Quality Assurance in General Dental Practice	Autumn 2004
Evidence-Based Care in General Dental Practice	Spring 2005

Quintessence Publishing Co. Ltd., London